A HIGHER STATE OF HEALTH

Cannabis Therapeutics for Women: Ancient Medicine to Flourish in the Modern World

Deirdra Martinez-Caso, MPH

Deirdra Martinez-Caso

To my parents, who march to the beat of their own drums and inspire me to pave my own path. To my husband, who is my biggest cheerleader and supports me through all my wild endeavors. To all those who fight to legalize cannabis and break the stigma, I am highly grateful.

CONTENTS

INTRODUCTION

Cannabis, also known as Marijuana, is making a comeback.

Prior to the 1920s, Cannabis was used medicinally and for manufactured goods like paper and clothes made of hemp. It was a valuable crop throughout the United States.

I didn't know this growing up. I was told there was a "War on Drugs" and that people who used them were criminals. Cannabis was labeled as "Gateway Drug" that lead to more lethal addictive drugs like cocaine or heroin. Sure, I experimented as a teenager as a form of rebellion and to feel accepted by my peers. What I didn't know then that I know now is that we've been fed myths about this therapeutic plant and that it could be an ally in health and healing.

From years of being in and out of doctors offices, I learned that health systems in the United States today need an upgrade. The emphasis is on treating the symptoms rather than the root cause. Health in the US is big business and it's more valuable for these companies to keep us sick than to help us thrive.

After getting my masters degree in public health, I was determined to make an impact in wellness. The best way was through prevention but unfortunately that just isn't sexy enough to be popular. Instead, I did most of my work in the fitness industry as a personal trainer working with women who wanted to lose weight. I had myself experienced my own body transformation. What I saw though was that as soon as something stressful happened in their lives, they would revert back to their old behaviors and gain the weight back again.

In our modern society, we're pushed to the brink of exhaustion in a culture that perpetuates a "work hard play hard" mindset. Mental illness and stress are making people physically sick. We're now suffering from many chronic stress related health problems like obesity, pain, insomnia, and depression. In this book we'll dive deeper into this and why we need to work at a deeper level.

When we turn to our health systems, we're desperate for answers and relief. We've become dependent on "experts" and "quick fixes." I realized that a lot of these diets and fitness programs that I followed and put my clients on were also "quick fixes." They were not helping my clients manage their health at a deeper level where they could sustain their results long term. Unfortunately, when we rely on these "quick fixes," we lose touch with our own innate healing ability and detach from the natural resources available, like plants.

As you read this book, you'll uncover the pervasive myths and mistakes that exist around Cannabis. For example, criminalizing cannabis is a business in and of itself. Not only does it feed the criminal system, but it also continues to allow pharmaceutical companies to make billions of dollars.

Although this book is written for women, it is useful for men as well. There are sections that address women's health and I share my story from a female's perspective. This book is rich in information that both men and women will find valuable.

I became inspired to write this book to share my journey of transforming my health with a cannabis inclusive lifestyle. After years of battling stress, anxiety, obesity, depression, and pain, I tried just about everything to find relief. It wasn't until I started using Cannabis therapeutically where I achieved a higher state of health.

Now that legalization is happening across the nation, it is important to get the education you need to be able to make the best choices. Cannabis is complex and there is a lot of information available, so much so that it might feel overwhelming to learn about it. This book provides facts and resources in a clear way so that you have a positive experience exploring cannabis for yourself.

I'll also share with you my Cannabis Therapeutics model that provides the foundation for getting the best results.

We now have the opportunity to medicate naturally in which we take our health back into our own hands.

CHAPTER 1 - GETTING UNSTUCK WITH CANNABIS

I learned about the value of cannabis after a long journey involving an eating disorder, substance abuse, chronic pain, and mental illness. I tried diets, abstinence programs, prescription pills, and just about anything that would offer me a quick fix to solve my problems. Nothing seemed to work long term. I felt broken and stuck. What lifted me out of that funk was pursuing a new way of healthy living that included cannabis.

Looking back, I always had an obsessive, compulsive, and anxious personality. There was no middle ground for me. It was all or nothing. I had extreme highs and lows, either resenting the past or fearing the future. Although I desired balance and inner peace, I was overtaken by constant cravings for food, drugs, alcohol, love, and validation.

First it was food. My gateway drug was McDonalds. By eight years old, I was eating super-sized Big Macs and 20-piece chicken nugget meals. On my 13th birthday, I weighed 190 pounds.

Although I didn't realize it at the time, I was already using food to help me cope with stressors at

home. My parents were divorced. My mother was a single parent who struggled financially to make ends meet. My father was in and out of rehab. I was sexually abused and experienced neglect. Life was not easy, and I developed a habit of using food to ease the pain and discomfort I felt. Of course, the eating made it worse. I felt even more disgusted with myself and was riddled with shame. I hated my body. It never really felt part of me, but rather like an object I had to drag around, the source of ridicule. Needless to say, I was bullied throughout elementary and middle school. When I was 15, I went on my first crash diet of eating nothing but low-fat frozen foods and running five miles a day. I was determined not to start high school as a fat girl.

My solution to the disgust I felt at my own body was to inflict ultra-strict diets on myself. As I said, all or nothing. I would swing grotesquely between binge eating everything I could lay my hands on followed by virtually nothing for days, sometimes weeks. Perversely the diets often made me feel better, at least mentally, as they allowed me to regain some measure of control and punish myself.

As I grew older, my addictive personality pushed out beyond just food. I introduced binge drinking and party drugs to the mix. Unsurprisingly, that led to men and sex in a futile attempt to validate my worth.

By my mid-20s, my drinking was out of control. Happy hours and clubbing became my release after working a job that I felt overwhelmed in and undervalued. I was too afraid to quit and so I distracted myself with drinking.

Alcohol was fun and worked until it became a problem. There were car accidents, fights, and one-night stands. Within the span a week, a series of events happened that made me open my eyes to "the rock bottom" I was in. I wrecked my car trying to make an illegal turn into a Wendy's fast food restaurant. It was the middle of the night, I was drunk, and I didn't realize there wasn't an actual drive-through entrance. I stopped at the curve and got hit by oncoming traffic. Luckily, I didn't get a DUI. While out partying, I got in a fight with a friend who ended up leaving me at the bar, forcing me to call another friend to pick me up. I also hooked up with a few different men, because in my mind that made me desirable.

It was that last night with a guy I met at a bar that triggered something. He took me back to his place where we did lines of coke and proceeded to have sex all night. The next morning, I found another woman's underwear in his bed. I tried to brush it off as a joke, slinging the G-string at him, but there was a disgusting, dark feeling deep inside. I thought, "I'm nothing to this guy. What if I end up with some sort of STD?"

When I met with my friends for brunch the next day, I was done talking about my escapades with men. I was ashamed and embarrassed. They were tired of it too because my stories always ended up the same. I knew that all the suffering I was experiencing was a result of my drinking, but I still couldn't stop.

The worst day of my life was when I walked into an Alcoholics Anonymous meeting for the first time. Don't get me wrong: these groups have helped millions of people, including my dad. But I felt utterly defeated. How had I got to this?

I'll never forget that first meeting. It was in the back of a coffee house in Santa Monica. The meeting room looked more like a small theatre. There was a stage with rows of red velvet theatre seats. The lights were dim. No one was on stage as if the audience was the actual show. As people went around the room sharing their stories, it was a real-life drama of overcoming adversity. I sat in the back row and couldn't stop crying.

The meeting was about to wrap up when the secretary said, "Any last burning desires?"

Something inside of me propelled me to raise my hand as if to save myself from a life sentence of self-destruction from holding my feelings inside. Weeping uncontrollably, I said, "I can't stop. I feel as if it's only a matter of time that something really bad is going to happen to me or someone else because of my drinking. I've been lucky so far but had too many close calls. My luck is bound to run out soon and I'm scared. I don't know what to do, so I came here."

There, I said it. I took a deep breath. Everyone was staring at me and collectively they took a deep breath. At the end of the meeting, several women approached me offering me their phone numbers. I felt weird. I didn't even know these women. Why would I call them? Why would they want me to call them? As if she could read my mind, a woman put her arm around me and said, "Let us love you until you can learn to love yourself."

The worst day of my life also turned out to be the beginning of my healing. It was a blessing.

At that moment I realized that I didn't really know what love was and I certainly didn't know how to love myself.

For five years, I was clean and sober. I attended AA meetings regularly and explored other 12-step programs like Overeaters Anonymous and Co-dependents Anonymous. I really cleaned up my life, but I was still suffering physically.

There is a phrase in the yoga community: the issues live in the tissues. I didn't realize it then, but all my unprocessed negative emotions and childhood trauma had lodged in my body and was manifesting in the form of back pain.

An increasing body of evidence demonstrates how the increased allostatic load associated with PTSD is also associated with physical issues in the form of chronic musculoskeletal pain, hypertension, hyperlipidemia, obesity, and cardiovascular disease.[1]

When I was drinking heavily, I hadn't noticed the physical pain I was in. When I got sober, the physical pain was all I could think about. I'd tried every doctor and treatment possible. Nothing helped. Surgery seemed like the only option left, but before that, I was referred to a psychiatrist first.

When I met with the psychiatrist, I was shocked when he said, "It's all in your head." I was diagnosed with anxiety at the age of 27. I didn't even know what that meant. It was the first time I learned that my thoughts and emotions had a direct effect on my body. My back pain was not rooted in physical injury but emotional repression, mental stress, and unhealed trauma.

The psychiatrist prescribed Prozac, which I thought was odd because I wasn't depressed. He explained that although it was an antidepressant, it had positive results for those with anxiety. I was desperate for relief and I trusted my doctor, so I agreed to the treatment.

Up until then, I lived with chronic stress and undiagnosed anxiety. I realized later that all my "bad habits" like overeating, binge drinking, and sleeping around were all my attempts to self-medicate my mental and emotional distress.

I am not the only one.

According to the Substance Abuse and Mental Health Services Association, an estimated 47.6 million adults aged 18 or older (19.1 percent) had a mental illness in 2018. An estimated 9.2 million adults aged 18 or older had a co-occuring mental illness and at least one substance use disorder in 2018.[2]

It's normal and common in our modern Western society to take pills for pain relief. I must admit, those first few months on Prozac were amazing. The back pain was gone, and I felt a sense of calm that I had never experienced before. I was focused and clear-headed.

There's no such thing as a quick fix, though. About six months later, I became depressed. It was a side effect of Prozac. I felt numb.

Having been a sensitive young woman, I felt terribly empty not feeling any emotion whatsoever. In an effort to feel something again, my binge eating disorder got out of control and my weight ballooned.

Quick fixes promise instant relief but downplay the long-term negative side effects. It's also simply putting a Band-Aid on the root cause of the pain.

The human mind and body are inextricably linked together. What impacts our mind impacts our body and vice versa. Our environment also impacts our physiological system. Everything is interwoven in a holistic balance. Chronic stress can create an imbalance in which the system begins to break down. This can manifest as physical or mental health problems. In my case, it was both.

This sense of connection and balance makes sense. When you're about to give a really important presentation, your heart starts to race. When you go out for a run, the body starts to sweat. There is a physiological response to your environment that keeps you in balance so that you can survive and thrive.

The issue is twofold. We may be disconnected and desensitized from our bodies and lack the ability to sense these subtle signals from within. Otherwise, we may be connected to our bodies but choose to distract or suppress the feeling that arise.

It became clear to me that my problem wasn't the back pain, anxiety, or even the depression that later emerged. Something far deeper was going on. There was a root source of the problem that I just couldn't sense.

The truth of our innate body wisdom and its power to restore health and healing is systematically dismissed and diminished by our culture and big pharmaceutical companies who want to pre-scribe *their* solution instead.

The narrative is simple—there is a pill we can take that will give us a quick fix to make the pain go away. Never mind that many of those so-called solutions are themselves addictive and come with a terrifying list of serious side effects. Whether it is a pill or a diet, these quick fixes may not provide a long-term solution.

Prozac only desensitized me even more from really tuning into what the deeper issue was. It was easier to stay numb and not feel what was happening in my life. Eventually this escapism led to depression.

When I told the doctor about my depression, his suggestion was to give me more pharmaceutical pills. That's when I knew it was time to look for an alternative solution.

At the time, a coworker was using Medical Marijuana (cannabis) as part of her cancer therapy. She told me how dispensaries offered cannabis to treat pain, anxiety, and depression. I was very interested. The only problem is that I was afraid of losing my sobriety. If I used cannabis as an alternative to Prozac, I wouldn't be accepted into Alcoholics Anonymous.

I was brought up thinking cannabis was a gateway drug and was afraid I would lose myself to drugs and alcohol again. However, it also didn't sit well with me that Prozac altered my state making me feel like a zombie—yet that was perfectly legal and socially acceptable. I also knew from experience that I had more challenges with food than I ever did with cannabis. Again, McDonald's was my gateway drug. I experimented with Marijuana as a kid, but it never amounted to anything more. Needless to say, I put a lot of thought into it.

I replaced my prescription antidepressants with cannabis, a plant that has been used for medicinal purposes for thousands of years. The earliest written accounts of cannabis used as medicine originated in China 4,700 years ago. [3]

One of the hardest things I had to do was tell my sponsor that I was using cannabis and tell my dad that I was no longer going to AA. Fortunately, they both were loving and accepting.

I had to find other resources for recovery that was inclusive of my cannabis use. Eventually, I found acceptance in the yoga community. Yoga is a group of spiritual, physical, and mental practices that originated in India. Holy men from India, called Sadhus, consume cannabis (also known as Bhang or Hashish) as part of their spiritual practice.

While using cannabis, I quit my stressful job and started my own fitness business. I turned my passion for nutrition and exercise into something that could support my livelihood. The Uplift Movement, my health and fitness company, evolved out of a desire to empower women in their wellness journey.

I continued to grow that business throughout my 30s, while using cannabis to manage my own anxiety. I became a yoga teacher and studied other healing modalities such as reiki, breathwork, and eating psychology. In that process, I healed my relationship with my body and food. No more body shaming or food restriction. Loving my body, even at its heaviest, freed me from the chronic stress of self-deprecation. The extra pounds naturally came off. My results, as well as my clients, started to improve as we went beyond diet and exercise by incorporating alternative healing therapies.

The challenges I experienced with my health were catalysts for change. They were wake up calls that I wasn't practicing self-love and self-care. I was overthinking which resulted in symptoms of chronic stress—chronic pain, addiction, and stubborn fat.

Cannabis was instrumental in my own health and healing, but I wasn't comfortable with sharing my experience with others. Unfortunately, due to stigma, safe access to cannabis as an alternative or complementary medicine is limited due to legalization issues.

I am an example of someone who uses cannabis and has a healthy, productive, and meaningful life. I went against the odds of relapse in traditional recovery. Although I use cannabis, my life is actually better than it's ever been and continues to evolve.

Today, at the age of 40, I'm married to the most wonderful man who loves me unconditionally. We're expecting our first baby (having no problems with fertility considering I used cannabis for many years). I operate my own wellness business while having a flourishing career in the cannabis industry. The relationships I have with my parents are the best they've ever been. No longer do I suffer from chronic back pain, addiction, depression, anxiety, or stubborn fat.

Through the practices I am going to share with you in this book, I've been able to create a higher state of health—one in which I've discovered newfound freedoms by living a balanced and authentic life.

Dr. Gabor Mate, an addiction expert and author of *In the Realm of Hungry Ghosts, Close Encounters with Addiction*, says, "Healing is not about 'staying away from something bad,' but about 'living a life led by positive values and intentions.'"

Cannabis can play an important role in health and healing. Don't buy into the myths, stigmas, and prejudices. Legalization is having a hugely positive impact on our society, health, and culture. I can share products with my loved ones, feeling completely confident that they are safe and effective.

My mom uses cannabis to treat her carpal tunnel syndrome, diabetes, and insomnia. My grandma loves her "cookies de medicina" and body creams to treat her arthritis. Some of my friends who want to drink less alcohol are finding a healthier alternative with cannabis beverages, as there are no calories or hangovers.

Cannabis is going mainstream and consumers need to be educated in order to make responsible choices. In order to do that, let's drop the stigma and rise up to the medicinal potential this therapeutic plant offers.

I wrote this book to share my health journey using cannabis as complementary medicine to treat my health issues. It will also provide resources and support on how to use cannabis therapeutically, so that the experience is safe and effective. Make sure to speak with a doctor before engaging in Cannabis use. For a network of doctors who support cannabis visit: https://www.cannabisclinicians.org/find-a-cannabis-doctor/ or https://thereleafinstitute.com/

This is not meant to promote cannabis as a magic pill. Instead, we'll dive into learning more about this medicinal plant and how lifestyle factors like nutrition, movement, and stress management all play a valuable role in healing.

CHAPTER 2 - BROKEN SYSTEMS

Back when I suffered from anxiety, my mind was like a loose cannon, shooting thoughts all day, every day. My emotions followed the same chaos. I was constantly concerned about my weight, finding my future husband, growing my career, and making money. What I didn't know then that I know now, is that a busy mind is stressful and left untamed, it can cause serious health issues.

It shouldn't have taken me so long to get help, but there is a stigma against mental illness. In minority cultures especially, we don't talk about stress. It's considered a sign of weakness. Our culture is also influenced by big pharmaceutical companies in which prescription pills are the trusted source for treatment, even if they're addictive or come with serious side effects. Yet, access to holistic medicine like cannabis is not only limited, but shamed.

It wasn't the weight gain, back pain, anxiety, or even the depression that was the real problem. Those were all just symptoms of a deeper issue. I realized that I needed to stop looking for the perfect diet, doctors, or trainers.

I needed to ask different questions—questions like:

"Why was it so hard to ease my restless mind?"

"Why was it so hard to control my emotions?"

"Why does it feel like no matter how hard I try, I can't sustain inner peace?"

"How can I heal naturally?"

These became the questions that guided my quest to uncovering healthier coping mechanisms and using plant medicine as a tool for elevating my wellbeing and happiness. I knew that if I didn't heal myself, everything would fall apart. I had been in the dark about stress for so long that it was extremely difficult to recognize and heal it. It is no surprise that eventually my body's pains became louder and louder as a sort of wake-up call.

It wasn't just a problem for me. It's an issue within our Western society.

"Stress in America continues to escalate and is affecting every aspect of people's lives—from work to personal relationships to sleep patterns and eating habits, as well as their health," says psychologist Russ Newman, PhD, JD, APA executive director for professional practice. "We know that stress is a fact of life and some stress can have a positive impact, however, the high stress levels that many Americans report experiencing can have long-term health consequences, ranging from fatigue to obesity and heart disease."[4]

In 2017, the American Psychological Association, reported the top 3 causes of stress in the US[5]:

1. (63%) Future of our Nation - Mass Shootings, War, Health Care (As of March 2020, we can probably add a Pandemic)
2. (62%) Job Pressure - Coworker tension, Bosses, Work Overload
3. (61%) Money - Loss of Job, Reduced Retirement, Medical Expenses

I have different sources of stress today than I had when I was 27. Ten years later, I'm less concerned about finding a husband (I'm now married) and more concerned about the state of our country. That's not a surprise, as culture influences our lives, from how we think to what we value.

As I write this today in May 2020, we're in the midst of a pandemic and protests that are triggering fears in all three of these categories. Approximately 150,000 people have died due to complications from COVID-19. The unemployment rate is at 11 percent, almost at the levels of The Great Depression. Non-essential workers are required to work from home where they may also be challenged to home school their children at the same time because schools are closed. Luckily, cannabis is classified as an essential business and available for purchase. On May 25, George Floyd, a 46-year-old Black man was murdered by white policemen holding a knee to his neck for 8 minutes and 46 seconds. It sparked protests all over the world demanding justice and change in systemic racism. Alongside the protests are riots and unrest with military forces being brought into cities to control the disorder. It feels as if we're on the brink of a civil war.

The media propagates so much fear that we eventually become desensitized. In other words, stress becomes normalized. Although 28 percent of Americans say that they're managing their stress very well, 77 percent report experiencing physical symptoms and 73 percent report psychological symptoms related to stress in the past month. Four in ten or 43 percent say they overeat or eat unhealthy foods to manage stress. Those who drink (39 percent of Americans) or smoke cigarettes (19 percent of Americans) were also more likely to engage in these unhealthy behaviors during periods of high stress. 43 percent of Americans report watching TV for more than two hours a day to cope with stress.[4]

How effective are we really at managing our stress? Considering those statistics, it doesn't seem like we are managing effectively at all when our coping mechanisms are leading to additional health problems.

There is a strong mind body connection. When we experience stress, there is a physiological response for survival. The sympathetic nervous system gets triggered, firing off stress hormones like adrenaline and cortisol. We subconsciously prepare for "fight, flight, or freeze" mode. When this happens, heart rate increases, breathing becomes shorter and more rapid, blood flow moves from the internal organs to the outer limbs. Metabolism, digestion, cognitive thinking, immune and cardiovascular systems are all compensated. When we experience chronic stress, these biological systems suffer, which leads to health problems and diseases like autoimmune issues, heart attacks, stubborn fat, constipation, insomnia, and more. It only gets worse when engaging in any of the unhealthy coping mechanisms.

One of the challenges I've faced as a fitness trainer and health coach is that most people want a quick fix. Women will often approach me and say, "Why can't I lose weight even though I eat healthy and exercise?" During our discovery sessions, we dig a little deeper and come to find out they're also not sleeping, constipated, exhausted, anxious, overwhelmed, and haven't had sex in months (even years!). They assume that I will suggest some sort of "diet hack" like a cleanse or supplement. Maybe in the past, their health problems resolved temporarily from one of those "hacks," but then they struggled to sustain their results. The truth is, women's health is much more complex than any single diet can solve. Because women are highly intuitive, stress can have much more of an impact on their health than most people imagine.

Women are more likely to experience more physical signs of stress compared to men.[6] The symptoms of stress include:

- **Headaches and migraines.** When you are stressed, your muscles tense up. Long-term tension can lead to headache, migraine, and general body aches and pains. Tension-type headaches are common in women.[7]

- **Depression and anxiety.** Women are almost twice as likely as men to have symptoms of depression.[8] Women are more likely than men to have an anxiety disorder, including post-traumatic stress disorder, panic disorder, or obsessive-compulsive disorder.[9]

- **Heart problems.** High stress levels can raise your blood pressure and heart rate. Over time, high blood pressure can cause serious health problems, such as stroke and heart attacks. Younger women with a history of heart problems especially may be at risk of the negative effects of stress on the heart.[10]

- **Upset stomach.** Short-term stress can cause stomach issues such as diarrhea or vomiting. Long-term stress can lead to irritable bowel syndrome (IBS), a condition that is twice as common in women as in men.[11] Stress can make IBS symptoms such as gas and bloating worse.

- **Obesity.** The link between stress and weight gain is stronger for women than for men.[12] Stress increases the amount of a hormone in your body called cortisol, which can lead to overeating and cause your body to store fat.

- **Problems getting pregnant.** Women with higher levels of stress are more likely to have problems getting pregnant than women with lower levels of stress. Also, not being able to get pregnant when you want to can be a source of stress.[13]

- **Decreased sex drive.** Women with long-term stress may take longer to get aroused and may have less sex drive than women with lower levels of stress. While not surprising, at least one study found that women with higher stress levels were more distracted during sex than other women.[14]

- **Aging and Menopause.** Frequently reported symptoms include difficulty sleeping, night sweats, headaches, hot flushes or flashes, vaginal dryness, forgetfulness, dizzy spells, stiff joints, feeling tense or nervous, feeling blue or depressed, and irritability.[15] Attitudes toward aging and menopause, perceived stress, and income were related to intensity of symptoms.[16]

While these health symptoms may cause discomfort and pain,

many women struggle to find long term relief. Although Americans recognize that stress has a negative impact on their health, they may lack the motivation to make lifestyle and behavior changes. Only 35 percent of Americans report that they would modify their behavior following the diagnosis of a chronic condition.[4]

Sound familiar? You come home from a stressful day at the office. You've been rocking your keto diet all week. You go into the kitchen to grab a light snack and see the kids' chips or cookies. Hmmmm. You think, "I'll just have one." Before you know it, you're plopped on the couch with the whole bag and mindlessly eating while watching TV. Then you feel so guilty for cheating on your diet that you vow to start all over again on Monday and work-out extra hard on the weekend.

Maybe food isn't your thing. Maybe it's alcohol? Shopping? Screen time? Sex? Work?

If you're like me, you've developed a habit of using a substance or engaging in a behavior to distract from pain or discomfort. We develop these habits from our early childhood. When I was a little girl, my parents treated me to a McDonalds Happy Meal whenever I was upset (I had that supersized by the way). It was no fault of their own. It's a cultural norm to not talk about emotions. As a society, we frown upon pain. Biologically, it's in our nature to seek pleasure and avoid pain. It's easier to use pleasurable substances or behaviors to numb the discomfort of stress than to actually feel the uncomfortable experience.

Digging deeper into our pain may seem daunting and may even trigger fear, shame, or guilt. We know it's not easy to do transformative work, so it's no surprise that people would rather look for a "magic pill" or "quick fix" without really addressing the core problem -- the root of stress. Here are a few common chronic health problems linked to stress where individuals are being exploited.

- **Obesity** - Where 31 percent of Americans are obese, 48 percent of American believe that it is because of diet.[17] It is no surprise that we have a $50 billion dollar weight loss industry fueled on easing the pain of being overweight with a quick-fix diet.[18] The reality is that there is a strong correlation between obesity and mental illness. Among those who suffer from eating disorders:
  - Alcohol and other substance abuse disorders are four times more common than in the general populations[19]
  - Depression and other mood disorders co-occur quite frequently[20]
  - There is a markedly elevated risk for obsessive-compulsive disorder[21]

- **Anxiety & Depression** - When it comes to treating mental health, the Center for Disease Control found that one in five adults is now taking at least one psychotropic medication. In 2010, Americans spent more than $16 billion on anti-psychotics and $11 billion on antidepressants.[22] There is also concern that children are being overmedicated. The latest estimate from the National Center for Health Statistics reports that 7.5 percent of U.S. children between ages six and 17 were taking medication for "emotional or behavioral difficulties" in 2011-2012.[23]

- **Chronic Pain** - America has declared a Public Health emergency on Opioid addiction. Roughly 21 to 29 percent of patients prescribed opioids for chronic pain misuse them.[24] Between 8 percent and 12 percent develop an opioid use disorder. An estimated 4 percent to 6 percent who misuse prescription opioids transition to heroin. About 80 percent of people who use heroin first misused prescription opioids. Opioid overdoses increased 30 percent from July 2016 through September 2017 in 52 areas in 45 states.[25]

If these treatments are expensive and ineffective, then why are they socially acceptable and promoted? One reason is that big pharmaceutical businesses have big ties (that is, money) for lobbying and marketing, which influences people's perception.

However, there is a growing demand for holistic alternative treatment for chronic stress and its associated symptoms, specifically with plant medicine psychedelics like cannabis, psilocybin (magic mushrooms), and ayahuasca. The Multidisciplinary Association of Psychedelic Studies (MAPS) is a non-profit organization that aims to provide research in the field of Psychedelics as medicine. As of 2020, MAPS is leading the research on using MDMA to treat PTSD with great success and are in the third phase of clinical trials. In addition, the added lifestyle changes promoted by Eastern medicine like yoga and meditation can help with maintaining long term results.

These plant medicines have played a vital role in my own personal health journey. Traditionally, these plants are used in spiritual ceremonies with trained practitioners (such as shamans, curanderos, and medicine men/women). Although they may be effective, they may be difficult to find due to laws and regulations in the west. However, cannabis is defying those odds and becoming more accessible for mainstream use.

As of February 2020, cannabis is legal for medical use in 33 states, yet there is still a stigma around this plant and its users. It is more socially acceptable to use pharmaceutical drugs rather than cannabis, even though it's been used as a medicine for thousands of years. Because cannabis is federally illegal, the research that people need to make educated decisions is limited. Instead, consumers end up relying on anecdotal accounts, friend referrals, and the internet.

I've often heard of the growth of the legal cannabis industry in the US as being referred to as "The Wild West." Regulations are still confusing for manufacturers, suppliers, and consumers. Companies with products, especially in the CBD market, are making health claims that cannot be proved or supported. Knock-off products that industry professionals often refer to as "snake oil" that are flooding the CBD market. It makes it overwhelming, confusing, difficult and challenging to explore cannabis as an alternative or complementary medicine.

This leads us to three problems:

1. Americans are self-medicating their chronic stress and its associated symptoms with powerful substances and self-sabotaging behaviors which may be causing additional health problems.

2. Pharmaceuticals are costly and may be over prescribed with side effects that leave the patient dependent on more expensive medications.

3. Cannabis may be effective in treating chronic stress and its health-related symptoms but stigma, lack of research and education creates a barrier to access.

It's time for a paradigm shift in how we address health and the opportunities that alternative therapies like cannabis can provide. In America, we have the right to bear arms with guns that kill people. Isn't it hypocritical to not provide the same right to self-medicate with natural plant-based drugs? Sugar, alcohol, guns, and automobiles can kill people. However, none of those are illegal. We can reclaim our freedom and exercise our right to alternative health treatments.

Research is growing with universities like UCLA providing research and resources available at https://www.uclahealth.org/cannabis/. In addition, countries like Israel are paving the way in cannabis therapeutics. There are now more opportunities for higher states of health. Let's explore.

CHAPTER 3 – WHAT IS CANNABIS THERAPEUTICS?

The Uplift Movement started as a fitness brand that evolved to include cannabis therapeutics, a holistic lifestyle system that can provide relief and freedom from chronic stress health issues. By using plant therapy combined with fitness, nutrition, and stress management, we are elevate happiness naturally while putting health back into own hands.

Cannabis therapeutics works by addressing the endocannabinoid system (ECS), one of the most important physiological systems involved in maintaining health. It was discovered in 1992, at the Hebrew University in Jerusalem by Dr. Lumir Hanus and American researcher Dr. William Devane.

The ECS is under research and may be involved in regulating physiological and cognitive processes, including fertility, appetite, pain-sensation, mood, sleep, and memory.[26] The ECS is composed of endocannabinoids, receptors, and enzymes.

For those interested in diving more into the science of the ECS, download my Cannabis Health Handbook at https://www.deirdramartinez.com/cannabishealthhandbook

In a nutshell, our body produces its own chemical compounds (endocannabinoids) that mimic the chemical compounds found in cannabis (phytocannabinoids or cannabinoids for short). We also have a receptor system that works like a "lock and key" with these endocannabinoids and cannabinoids.

These endocannabinoids and their receptors are found throughout the body: in the brain, organs, connective tissues, glands, and immune cells. With its complex actions in our immune system, nervous system, and virtually all of the body's organs, the endocannabinoids are literally a bridge between body and mind.[27]

The ECS works as a neuromodulator, sustaining balance in the body (also known as homeostasis). For example, when we cut ourselves, the body naturally starts to repair that wound. There's a natural movement towards restoration and balance. Although this area of research is quite controversial, several phytocannabinoids, especially cannabidiol (CBD), have been suggested to exert beneficial effects in various pathological conditions, including inflammation, cancer, addiction and epilepsy.[28]

CBD is now scientifically proven to reduce seizures. In 2017, the FDA approved Epidiolex, a pharmaceutical drug derived from cannabis CBD to treat epilepsy.[29] This sparked more research on the therapeutic benefits of cannabis. CBD and THC (tetrahydrocannabinol) are now being studied for chronic stress symptoms like pain, anxiety, depression, insomnia, autoimmune, and even stubborn fat.[30]

In cannabis therapeutics, we work with both the nervous system and ECS while optimizing their functionality with lifestyle enhancements. These two biological systems affect the efficiency of digestion, metabolism, immunity, endocrine, muscular and cardiovascular systems. When it comes to the nervous system, adopting a baseline of parasympathetic mode provides a calm internal environment. The Parasympathetic Nervous System (PNS) is often referred to "Rest and Digest," which is optimal for healing, health, and vitality. This in effect allows the ECS to restore balance in the body on a continual basis without impairment from stress.

When we perceive a threat, like if we're worried about the state of the nation or stressed out about the security of our jobs, money, or health, then the nervous system gets triggered to be in Sympathetic mode (SNS) which is "fight, flight, or freeze." This prepares the body for self-preservation in case that threat becomes a reality. Stress hormones are activated, tensing muscles around the shoulders, jaw, and back. Heart rate increases, moving blood flow away from the internal organs and towards the outer limbs so that the body can quickly react. Digestion, immunity, and metabolism shut down in order to preserve energy for survival. Chronic stress keeps the body in this constant survival mode and eventually leads to physical and mental illness, disease, pain, and even substance abuse disorders like stress eating or binge drinking.

Cannabinoids THC is one of at least 113 cannabinoids found in cannabis and provides the psychoactive effect. THC also mimics the body's own naturally occurring endocannabinoids as well as anandamide (known as "the bliss molecule") which enhances the feeling of euphoria. CBD is another cannabinoid that mimics the endocannabinoid 2-AG. CBD and 2-AG are involved in the regulation of the immune system and pain management.[31]

Chronic stress impairs both the nervous system and ECS which can lead to chronic health problems like mental illness (including anxiety, depression, and ADHD), autoimmune disease, digestive and metabolic disorders, pain, and insomnia. Cannabinoids act as neuromodulators for a variety of processes including motor learning, appetite, and pain sensation, among other cognitive and physical processes. Other examples of neuromodulators include dopamine and serotonin.

Cannabis therapeutics restores the body's natural ability to heal and perform optimally. Through a holistic program, we utilize meditation, nutrition, and fitness to reduce stress and enhance wellbeing. We complement this work with plant medicine, like cannabis, which provides natural relief and therapeutic support.

I decided to treat my anxiety with cannabis back in 2010 when little research was available on the therapeutic benefits. I had to "wing it" and it was a bit sloppy for awhile. Little did I know that without the foundations of nutrition, fitness, and meditation, my cannabis use wasn't therapeutic; it was recreational. Big difference. Recreational is similar to drinking wine with friends. We do it for fun, socializing, relaxation, and also as a distraction. However, you run the risk of substance abuse and even addiction. Over time, I learned how to integrate the modalities that allowed me to gain the most benefit from this plant medicine without abuse. I will share those secrets with you now!

The Cannabis Therapeutics Model

The Uplift Movement is the platform for cannabis therapeutics and was founded on three principles: Education, Elevation, and Empowerment.

1. **Education** - We provide research-based cannabis health education that includes holistic health practices such as yoga, meditation, fitness, and nutrition.
2. **Elevation** - We support each other in the process of transcending health challenges and moving beyond suffering.
3. **Empowerment** - We strengthen women's confidence, so that they can take back their health.

In addition, The Uplift Movement cannabis therapeutics is supported by four healthy lifestyle practices:

1. Mindfulness Meditation
2. Movement
3. Nutrition
4. Cannabis

In this model, elevating health and happiness comes from a holistic approach that goes beyond treating the symptoms alone. By combining meditation, movement, nutrition, and cannabis, there is attention brought to balancing both the nervous system and the ECS. When brought into balance, these systems work synergistically to achieve optimal function of various other systems like immune, digestion, metabolism, and more. When clients incorporate these healthy lifestyle practices, they experience improvements in chronic health conditions such as insomnia, obesity, autoimmune, digestive disorders, and pain management.

Mindfulness Meditation

Based on Zen Buddhism, the practice of Mindfulness Meditation is a way of life that brings the practitioner into the present moment. This type of meditation is known to calm the mind, reduce stress, and improve overall health. Jon Kabat Zinn brought this form of meditation to the West and teaches Mindfulness-Based Stress Reduction (MBSR). Studies have shown benefits against an array of conditions like irritable bowel syndrome, fibromyalgia, psoriasis, anxiety, depression, and post-traumatic stress disorder.[32]

This eight-week practice is intended to help the student become aware of the narratives that constantly run through their mind. Ongoing thinking has an impact on the body, especially when those thoughts are negative or worrisome. Ruminating about the past or obsessing about the future can actually trigger a chronic stress response in the body where our baseline is in the SNS "flight or fight." Through the techniques learned in MBSR, we develop tools to overcome stress and restore inner peace. The result is a reduction in chronic stress health problems. While chronic stress can create an imbalance on your ECS, a highly-tuned ECS can protect you from the detrimental effects of stress.[33]

Movement

An exercise-induced altered state of consciousness has long been appreciated by endurance athletes.[34] I myself was a marathon runner for about five years. This was at a time where I was obsessed with weight loss and I believed running marathons would help me manage my weight. Although I didn't lose the weight as I hoped, I did experience the "runner's high." The runner's high has been described subjectively as pure happiness, elation, a feeling of unity with one's self and/or nature, endless peacefulness, inner harmony, boundless energy, and a reduction in pain sensation.[34] These subjective descriptions are similar to the claims of distorted perception, atypical thought patterns, diminished awareness of one's surroundings, and intensified introspective understanding of one's sense of identity and emotional status made by people who describe drug or trance states.[34]

Recent data shows that endurance exercise activates the endocannabinoid system.[35] Long-distance running is not for everyone, especially if you're someone who suffers from anxiety or chronic pain. I don't run like that anymore. In addition, any type of endurance high-intensity exercises may have the opposite effect on the nervous system triggering SNS. Moderate intensity exercises like walking, dancing and weight training can be better alternatives for those with an overactive SNS. In addition, incorporating restorative exercises like yin yoga and Tai-Chi can activate the PNS which is calming, relaxing, and healing.

Get a free class pass to take my livestream online workouts

plus get access to my on demand video library at https://www.deirdramartinez.com/freeclasspass

Nutrition

Nutrition is more than cutting calories or restricting certain foods on a trendy diet. It means changing your relationship with food and body. Most women who are educated and well-resourced already know how to eat a healthy diet and yet there's still excuses like "I don't have enough time to cook" or "I'm too tired at the end of a day to deal with cooking."

There's also the issue that plagues many women, which is mindless eating. All too often, women are using food to cope with stress or provide pleasure. They can feel guilt and shame when they overeat or "cheat" and will use diets to try and gain control again. The stress of following a perfect diet becomes too much and they end up "cheating" again. It becomes a vicious yo-yo dieting cycle. Body weight development and maintenance are fundamental to maintain health and to promote longevity, while underweight, overweight, and specifically obesity in childhood, adolescence and adulthood are associated with adverse health consequences throughout the life course.[36]

Eating a Western diet packed with processed foods, sugars and unhealthy fats can create problems for your health and your waistline. These diets also negatively impact your endocannabinoid system. The endocannabinoid (eCBs), 2AG, controls your appetite (which is why THC can stimulate hunger), and Western diets can lead to increased production of eCBs in the intestine and circulatory system, making you hungrier.[37] Added to this problem is the finding that fat cells produce even more eCBs, which means that overweight people often have higher levels of eCBs stoking their hunger, making it harder to lose weight.[38]

Certain foods can help the endocannabinoid system function optimally, improve your health, and enhance the effectiveness of medicinal cannabis. A healthy ratio of omega-3 and omega-6 fatty acids can enhance the activity of the ECS.[39] Cacao powder contains three compounds that are structurally very similar to endocannabinoids.[40] These compounds can inhibit the breakdown of your body's own endocannabinoids, resulting in higher endocannabinoid levels. The content of cannabinoid-like compounds in chocolate varies widely and is highest in dark chocolate and raw cacao. Numerous herbs and teas contain compounds that can enhance the ECS. Turmeric, the yellow spice in curry powder, contains curcumin, which also raises endocannabinoid levels amongst numerous other health benefits.[41]

Cannabis is also fat soluble. When consuming cannabis as an edible, have it with a healthy fat like coconut oil, avocado, or peanut butter. It will help boost the effects.

Cannabis

In 2007, "The Godfather of Cannabis Research" Dr. Rapheal Mechoulam said, "Cannabinoids represent a medicinal treasure trove which waits to be discovered." Although it may be more socially acceptable to use straight CBD without THC, the full potential of the therapeutic benefits are found in the combination of both phytocannabinoids. All the various phytocannabinoids work synergistically providing an "entourage effect."

A 2016 study found that THC and CBD contents were the most important factor for optimizing symptom relief for a wide variety of health conditions.[42] From that same study, Dr. Jacob Miguel Vigil, associate professor in the Department of Psychology states, "Despite the conventional wisdom, both in the popular press and much of the scientific community that only CBD has medical benefits while THC merely makes one high, our results suggest that THC may be more important than CBD in generating therapeutic benefits. In our study, CBD appears to have little effect at all, while THC generates measurable improvements in symptom relief. These findings justify the immediate de-scheduling of all types of cannabis, in addition to hemp, so that cannabis with THC can be more widely accessible for pharmaceutical use by the general public."[45]

Cannabis can be consumed in a variety of methods including smoking, ingestibles, topicals, and sublinguals. The method of consumption should be determined based on the individual's health condition. There are also a variety of ratios of CBD to THC that you can find that make dosing easier and the experience more pleasant. For example, those that may be worried about getting "high" can take a 20:1 (CBD:THC) tincture which provides the entourage effect without impairing the consumer.

Discovering your therapeutic threshold is the basis of cannabis therapeutics. Too little and you won't experience any benefit, too much and you may experience an adverse effect. Keep in mind, cannabinoids can be biphasic, meaning that low and high doses can produce opposite effects. This is why it is critical to work with a guide or an expert to help identify the appropriate products, effective dosing, and track progress.

Microdosing is consuming 2mg or less throughout the day. Some find it very effective for symptom relief without causing impairment.

Remember to get a clearance from your cannabis friendly before exploring cannabis therapeutically. Many doctors are not trained in cannabis and may deter you from using it simply because they don't know enough. They may run the risk of losing their license if they give recommendations because cannabis is still federally illegal. It is strongly suggested to consult a cannabis-friendly doctor to clear whether your health conditions or other medications will not be negatively impacted by cannabis.

For Best Results

Unfortunately, many people who are using cannabis are not getting the full therapeutic benefits. That's because they bypass the lifestyle factors associated with enhancing the ECS. If you're not complementing your cannabis use with proper nutrition, fitness, and meditation, then it's really just recreational use. Recreational use is fine, but don't say, "I tried cannabis and it doesn't work."

Recently, I did a discovery session with someone interested in using cannabis to help calm their anxiety and help her lose weight. She told me she's been vaping and has been a consumer for years. Obviously, cannabis alone wasn't working.

When I explained to her that it took a lifestyle change that includes fitness, nutrition, and meditation, I was met with resistance and excuses.

Her: "I hate yoga. It's only for skinny bendy girls and I'm not like that."

Me: "I'm not a skinny bendy girl and I do yoga. There's many different kinds and we can find one that works for you."

Her: "I'd rather do kickboxing."

Me: "That's great. You can do kickboxing. However, for someone who suffers from anxiety incorporating more intense exercise is counterproductive. It will raise your stress hormones. We actually need to integrate more calming activities like walking or meditating."

Her: "Well, I can't meditate. I can't sit still. Besides, I need to burn more calories. I eat keto and so my nutrition is fine."

Me, "Ok. Keto works well for some individuals. However, do you find yourself cheating often? How long have you actually maintained your weight loss while on keto? We can work with you to create a way of eating that is all-inclusive and sustainable. You can still lose weight eating bread and carbs. Would you like me to show you how?"

We went on and on for quite some time. I got the impression she wasn't happy I didn't tell her what she wanted to hear. In this case, what she wanted was a recommendation for cannabis.

I understand the resistance because I was there too. We're a society that wants that "magic pill."

When I first replaced Prozac with cannabis, I thought the cannabis itself would be enough. I wanted to do things my way which was unfortunately filled with stress inducing activities. I over exercised with high intensity cardio classes. This was at the time where I was starting my fitness career. I was teaching up to 5 Zumba and spinning classes per day. My eating habits were extreme going back and forth between "competition dieting" (I literally competed in fitness competitions) and binge eating. I brushed off meditation and yoga as something I just didn't have time or patience for.

What ended up happening was that I became dependent on cannabis. Remember that cannabis is a powerful substance. As with sugar, we can develop a substance dependence on cannabis. I kept myself "high" on cannabis throughout most of that time because I didn't have the life structures to support balance and wellbeing.

The "universe" works in mysterious ways. I probably would have stayed stuck if it wasn't for an injury I got while teaching Zumba. I couldn't teach for months. I was forced to slow down and change my habits. On the brink of depression, I pushed myself to go to a yoga class because it was literally the only activity I could do. It was awkward and uncomfortable, but I was humbled to just be off the couch. I kept going back and slowly I fell in love with yoga.

That injury turned out to be the best thing that happened to me because it launched a new level of health transformation that I experienced from becoming a yoga teacher.

That challenge turned into a transformative experience. I had to let go of beliefs and habits that were sabotaging my wellbeing. I was able to learn and develop a new lifestyle that actually helped me thrive.

Plain and simple: don't expect cannabis to relieve your symptoms if you're not making the effort to change your lifestyle. The sooner you realize this, the faster you can take action and get better results.

Sure, products may try to influence you to think otherwise. You'll find these sorts of claims especially in the hemp CBD market because it's unregulated. Who doesn't want a "magic pill?" You can now smell the "BS" and avoid wasting your money on ineffective products. If you're going to make a good investment in high quality products, don't cut yourself short by not investing also in your diet, fitness, and stress management.

The bottom line is that it's an imbalance in your lifestyle that caused the issue in the first place, it's going to take getting back into balance in order to heal. Cannabis is a tool, not the cure.

Cannabis therapeutics is unique to every individual and requires a customized approach. At The Uplift Movement, we work together to customize your healthy lifestyle while supporting your journey with cannabis. We examine your specific health challenge and explore how cannabis can complement. Visit www.deirdramartinez.com to learn more or to book a free consultation.

Cannabis Therapeutics for Common Symptoms of Chronic Stress

Before exploring cannabis therapeutics, especially if you have a serious pre-existing health issue, talk to a doctor first.

What is shared in this section is based on personal experience and research. Remember that each individual is unique in which body composition, emotional health, and environment all play a role in one's healing. How one individual reacts to a certain type of cannabis strain may be different than the other person. So, use this as a general guide to start your journey and then consider working with a professional to customize your program and improve your results. Keep a journal to track your results.

Mindfulness meditations are located toward the end of the chapter for reference. You can also download free audio resources from https://www.deirdramartinez.com/freemeditations.

Anxiety

Mindfulness Meditation

Try a body scan. When we're experiencing anxiety, we tend to be too much in our heads. It's like we're constantly running a movie in our head where we lose connection to our body. A body scan is a great way to ground back into the body and get out of the chaos in the mind. There is intuitive intelligence in the body that we can tap into when our mind is overwhelmed making us feel lost or stuck. The result will be more clarity, relaxation, and restoration. The Uplift Movement offers an 8 Week Mindfulness Program: Elevated Thinking that will walk you through the process of incorporating mindfulness mindful in everyday life. Learn more at https://www.deirdramartinez.com/products.

Movement

Avoid high intensity cardio fitness classes such as spinning or HIIT because it can stimulate more of a stress response in the body. Instead, opt for walking, hiking, tai-chi, and yoga. If you can enjoy movement outdoors in nature, even better!

Nutrition

The ancient practice of Ayurveda is the sister science of yoga. It is an ancient Indian medical system that focuses on restoring balance in the body. One way it does that is through nutrition by incorporating foods like cooked hearty stews, root vegetables, warm meals, and teas can be grounding for individuals who suffer from anxiety. Dr. Deepak Chopra is a leader in Ayurveda and you can read more about Ayurveda visiting his website at https://chopra.com/articles/an-ayurvedic-approach-to-anxiety. Limit caffeine as well as it can be too strong a stimulant.

Cannabis

Avoid Cannabis with high levels of THC as this can aggravate anxiety and increase paranoia especially among new users. Consider strains that have higher levels of CBD or are balanced between CBD and THC. These strains include Harlequin, Charlotte's Web, and Cannatonic.

You can also find tinctures, vape carts, and capsules that are formulated in ratios (CBD:THC) high in CBD such as 20:1 or 10:1. In a formulation like a 20:1, there may be little to no feeling of the psychoactive effect of THC. However, there is a small amount of THC, which gives you the full-spectrum effect, thus providing a more therapeutic value.

Some individuals find benefit in taking small amounts throughout the day (a process called microdosing) while others experience a benefit from having cannabis once a day. This is something unique to each individual and to explore through a process of starting with once a day and then gradually increasing until desired effect. During the evening, cannabis indica strains can promote relaxation which can help with unwinding before bedtime. My favorite evening ritual to relax is having cannabis indica strain and doing a meditation or a yin yoga class.

Depression

Mindfulness Meditation
Try Loving Kindness Meditation. This meditation stimulates the body's natural ability to produce the mood-enhancing "love hormone," oxytocin. This chemical modulates social interactions and emotion. The more oxytocin, the greater sense of connection and wellbeing.

Movement
Stimulate anandamide (the bliss molecule) naturally through song and dance. Put on music you love and do housework while you sing and have an occasional dance break. Take that fun playlist with you and go on a brisk walk. Mix it up on some days and go

on a walk with a close friend. Take a dance class online or in person. Dancing boosts endorphins and stimulates joy naturally.

Nutrition

A diet high in sugar, processed foods, caffeine, and/or fast food can increase fatigue and feelings of depression. In addition, eating large heavy meals can promote the feeling of sluggishness. Take a good look at the quality and quantity of food you're consuming. If you have a sweet tooth, add more fruit and natural sweeteners such as honey or stevia. Try replacing coffee with dandelion tea or medium caffeine tea. Add more wholesome vegetables, grains, and proteins rather than processed foods. Have these in smaller quantities throughout the day like three to five small meals throughout the day as opposed to two large meals.

Beyond nourishment with diet, how do you nourish your emotional wellbeing? What activities nourish you? What relationships nourish you? Make a list and start to add these into your life on a daily or weekly basis.

Cannabis

There is a chemical compound in cannabis known as anandamide which is also known as the bliss molecule. Anandamide is also produced naturally in the body. However, stress can impair our endocannabinoid system limiting the amount of anandamide produced in the body. Cannabis can help bring the endocannabinoid system back into balance and aid in restoring anandamide levels. However, too much cannabis can also leave the body dependent on the substance for anandamide rather than producing its own. This is why it's important to not just rely on cannabis alone and to complement usage with the other structures listed in this model that boost anandamide naturally. That way cannabis is taken "as needed" and you won't develop a dependence.

Although every cannabis strain has a different interaction to each individual based on their own body chemistry, in general, strains that are sativa are known to promote feelings of euphoria and energy. Nowadays it may be difficult to find a true sativa strain, so you can also opt for a hybrid that is sativa dominant. Microdosing allows you to take smaller amounts throughout the day allowing more control of the way you want to feel.

Weight Gain

Mindfulness Meditation

Try mindful eating. This practice elevates our relationship with food and heals our relationship with the body. It involves switching from autopilot to eating with awareness in an open and nonjudgmental way. There is an evolution of understanding nourishment at a deeper level. This is also known as slow eating. Mindful eating allows you to enjoy food more while managing weight effortlessly.

Mindful Movement

Individuals may be holding on to weight for various reasons and the type of exercise you do can also have an effect. For those that are stressed, high-intensity movement is counterproductive and not recommended. Although the temptation is there to "sweat it out" or burn a ton of calories, the opposite effect may be happening in the nervous system in which these high intensity exercise classes will increase stress hormones and make it harder to lose weight.

In this case, try low- to moderate-intensity workouts like yoga and strength training. Yoga is excellent as it also includes strength training (with your own body weight) which helps burn fat in the long-term. Yoga also balances the nervous system reducing the stress hormones that cause weight gain.

Nutrition

When it comes to nutrition, most of us already know what to eat. The problem is that there are too many trendy diets out there promoting fast weight loss, and it is very tempting to jump on the bandwagon, especially if you feel heavy.

What I've learned after many years of studying nutrition and weight loss is that the solution is much simpler: we need to change our relationship with food and body. This is done through a mindful eating practice and reconnecting with your body's own intuition regarding nourishment. The body has the wisdom and ability to do things like give birth, pump blood, and digest a meal without us having to think about it. Stress can show up in many different ways around food such as "what should I eat" or "I shouldn't have eaten that." We can experience shame, guilt, and frustration all feelings that can perpetuate a cycle of unhealthy eating.

It's not just important to focus on what you're eating, but how, when, and why you're eating. Elevated Eating: turn unwanted eating habits into a healing transformation with food and body is a program through The Uplift Movement that helps you explore this deeper. Learn more at https://www.deirdramartinez.com/products.

Cannabis

You may have heard of the "munchies" when you consume Cannabis. That may deter you from exploring Cannabis because you're afraid of overeating. The munchies can happen from consuming too much THC, especially if you haven't developed a tolerance to THC. Long term Cannabis consumers (who developed a tolerance) will actually have a lower BMI. A 2011 study on obesity and cannabis, published in the *American Journal of Epidemiology*, concluded that obesity rates were lower in cannabis smokers than in nonusers. Those that consumed three or more times per week were 40 percent less likely to be obese than those with no cannabis use in the past 12 months.[43]

In order to avoid the munchies, you can build a tolerance safely through microdosing, which involves taking small amounts less than 2mg of THC throughout the day. Another hack is to drink plenty of fluids. A side effect of cannabis can be dry mouth, which may cause you to think that you're hungry when you're really just thirsty.

There is also growing research on another chemical compound found in cannabis called THCV which may work as an appetite suppressant. Popular strains high in THCV are Tangie, Girl Scout Cookies, and Durban Poison.

Insomnia

Mindfulness Meditation

Try a body scan before bedtime. What can keep us up at night is a racing mind that can't be turned off. This meditation provides the opportunity to draw awareness into the body which is more grounding and relaxing.

Mindful Movement

It is important to avoid external stimulation from things like the TV, internet, social media, emails, news, and anything else that could set your mind in a tailspin of thinking. Instead, integrate a Yin Yoga practice as part of your evening routine. This will relax the body, calm the nervous system, prepare your mind and body for sleep. Visit my YouTube channel at The Uplift Movement to enjoy a free Yin Yoga practice from the comfort of your own home.

Nutrition

Limit the amount of caffeine and sugar in your diet as these can stimulate a stress response in the body, which makes it difficult to fall asleep. As part of your evening routine, include a cup of chamomile tea which is a natural herbal sedative. You can also try other supplements such as melatonin or valerian.

Cannabis

Cannabis strains that are more indica dominant can be more relaxing and may help ease the body to rest especially when combined with meditation or Yin Yoga. A few popular strains for a good night's sleep are Granddaddy Purple and Northern Lights.

There is ongoing debate regarding a chemical compound in Cannabis known as CBN which may also help promote sleep. Strains that contain high levels of CBN include Blackberry and Bubblegum.

Substance Abuse

Mindfulness Meditation

You could try sitting meditation, body scan, loving kindness, and mindful eating. Substance abuse can be a coping mechanism for anxiety, depression, trauma, and pain. Therefore, a variety of meditations are effective here. Mindful eating can be particularly helpful as well as it involves consuming a substance into the body and being present with that experience.

Oftentimes, someone who experiences substance abuse has challenges with a few different substances. For example, I not only had a drinking problem at one time in my life, but I also had an issue with food. Others may have problems with smoking, drugs (pharmaceutical and recreational), caffeine, and/or sugar. Learning how to be present with uncomfortable sensations as they arise without trying to fix or change them is extremely powerful. That's exactly what we learn through these practices.

Mindful Movement

Mix up activity for a balanced and scheduled routine. Exercise produces endorphins that enhance mood and sense of wellbeing. Make sure to also include yoga as it is therapeutic for any underlying physiological issues that may be at the root of substance abuse such as trauma. Enhance the experience by joining fitness groups so that you develop relationships within a health promoting community. Replace happy hours or daily late-night glass of wine with a walk, group fitness class, or meditation.

Nutrition

For some of us, there may be substance abuse issues around food. Perhaps the struggle is with sugar, carbs, snack foods, fast food, or dairy. Although the temptation may be to completely omit these foods, a sort of abstinence, that may actually cause more binging in the future.

One of the best ways to improve nutrition here is through a mindful eating practice. You can also find the benefits extending beyond food and into other substances such as smoking or drinking. Learning how to be present with a substance in an open and nonjudgmental way can foster empowered choices rather than struggling with addictive narratives.

Cannabis

A limited number of preclinical studies suggest that CBD may have therapeutic properties on opioid, cocaine, and psychostimulant addiction, and some preliminary data suggest that it may be beneficial in cannabis and tobacco addiction in humans. Further studies are clearly necessary to fully evaluate the potential of CBD as an intervention for addictive disorders.[44]

Chronic Pain

Mindfulness Meditation

A body scan meditation could be helpful. Pain can be psychosomatic, which is where the mind can trigger more painful sensations in the body especially through negative thinking. Worrying about the pain, future pain, frustration about circumstances due to pain, anger, resentment, all of these thoughts and emotions can send signals to the body increasing the sensation of pain.

Being present with the body during this meditation teaches us how to be aware of the sensations in the body as they change. Part of this practice is the realization of impermanence. Pain changes as in everything else in life. When we accept this, there is a greater sense of inner peace.

Mindful Movement

Movement can be tricky when it comes to chronic pain. In one way, there can be a balancing act between strength building and recovery. Many times, chronic pain can be a result of a muscle imbalance and weak muscles. For example, lower back pain may result from a weak core. The muscles of the abdomen need strength training while the muscles of the back need stretching. In another way, the body may need full-on recovery in which no movement or gentle stretching is recommended.

Follow guidelines provided by a physical therapist and stick to the program they provide. Part of the problem when I speak with clients who suffer from chronic pain is that they don't follow the exercise program provided by their physical therapist. They may do it for a few days, lose interest and stop otherwise they do it occasionally. This will not help with the healing process but instead keep the problem lingering.

Do the exercises mindfully by doing them free of distraction. Focus on breathing and connecting with the body which means feeling the muscles that are working, in an open and non-judgmental way. Depending on the severity of pain, some find benefit and improvement through a hatha yoga practice. This is a type of yoga that emphasizes longer holds in poses for mind and body strengthening. There is also an emphasis on meditation using breathwork which can be therapeutic for health and wellbeing.

Nutrition

Chronic pain may also be related to the types of food within a diet especially if it is full of inflammatory foods like sugar, excessive alcohol, excessive meat and refined carbohydrates. Swap these foods for more wholesome plants, omega 3s, and antioxidants.

Pain can also be a result of dehydration. My muscles in my upper back tense up not only when I'm stressed but also when I'm dehydrated. The body is mostly made up of water. If you're not drinking enough, muscles and joints can become stiff. The National Academies of Sciences, Engineering, and Medicine determined that an adequate daily fluid intake is:

- About 15.5 cups (3.7 liters) of fluids for men
- About 11.5 cups (2.7 liters) of fluids a day for women

You'll need more water if you work out often, if you live in a hotter environment, and if you're pregnant.

Cannabis

Whole Cannabis flower is associated with greater pain relief than were other types of products, and higher tetrahydrocannabinol (THC) levels were the strongest predictors of analgesia and side effects prevalence.[45] Side effects may include dry mouth, drowsiness, dizziness, and paranoid thinking (typically with high levels of THC content). High CBD strains can be good for inflammation. Taken orally (tincture, capsule, edible) the effects can last four to eight hours. If chronic pain makes it difficult to sleep at night, a 1:1 (THC:CBD) oil or capsule at bedtime may help. Individuals also find relief from topicals (ointments/creams) that have a combination of THC and CBD. When taken topically, there is no psychoactive effect. My grandmother loves Apothecanna cream and CBD cookies from Dr. Norms for her arthritis. For PMS related pain, suppositories can give direct internal relief. CBD Alive and Foria offer suppositories. Use these in the evening before bed as there may be discharge.

Cannabis and Opioids

More than 11.5 million Americans reported misusing prescription opioids in 2016.[46] Prescription painkillers have also been linked to heroin use. For every five new heroin users, four started with prescription pills.[47] In 2017, The US department of Health & Human Services declared a Public Health emergency in response to this Opioid Crisis. The risks of Opioids include abuse, addiction, overdose, and death. Over 130 people die every day from Opioid related drug overdoses. An estimated 40% of opioid overdose deaths involved a prescription opioid.[48]

Cannabis, a non-lethal drug, that has been used in the treatment of chronic pain for thousands of years. The demand for alternative medicine is on the rise. A study in 2014 found significant decreases in opioid overdose deaths where states had legalized medical marijuana. On average, these states had a near-25 percent lower mortality rate from opioids than states without such laws, and this correlation strengthened the longer medical marijuana was legal.[49] Cannabinoids act synergistically with opioids and act as opioid sparing agents, allowing lower doses and fewer side effects from chronic opioid therapy.[50]

Autoimmune diseases

Mindfulness Meditation

Sitting meditation, body scan, and loving kindness are all useful options. A variety of mindfulness meditation will benefit this condition. Mindfulness meditation appears to be associated with reductions in proinflammatory processes, increases in cell-mediated defense parameters, and increases in enzyme activity that guards against cell aging.[51]

Mindful Movement

With autoimmune conditions, the nervous system is in constant fight-or-flight mode because the body as the body can be literally attacking itself. Yoga, specifically restorative yoga, is a great way to shift the nervous system to rest and relaxation where healing can take place. Yoga is also therapeutic in the sense that it restores security and safety (taking the body out of fight or flight) by strengthening the mind and body connection. Restorative yoga is gentle and accessible for all bodies.

Nutrition

Food allergies can trigger an autoimmune response. One way to determine if there are any food allergies is by doing an elimination diet. There are two phases:

- Elimination diet – remove these foods that are common for sensitivities for two or three weeks: nuts, corn, soy, dairy, citrus fruits, nightshade vegetables, wheat, foods containing gluten, pork, eggs and seafood.

- o   Keep a journal and track the body's response.
- Reintroduction – One by one begin to reintroduce each food for a period of 2-3 days. Keep track if there is any physical response such as:
  - o   Skin rash
  - o   Joint pain
  - o   Fatigue
  - o   Migraines and headaches
  - o   Digestive discomfort
  - o   Insomnia
  - o   Change in bowel movements
- If there is a reaction to one of the foods, there may be a food allergy. There are also tests available through a doctor to have it confirmed. Then experiment by eliminating that food item for a long period of time and notice if the symptoms subside.

Cannabis

The endocannabinoid system is involved in immunoregulation. Cannabinoids have been tested in several experimental models of autoimmune disorders such as multiple sclerosis, rheumatoid arthritis, colitis and hepatitis and have been shown to protect the host from the pathogenesis through induction of multiple anti-inflammatory pathways.[52] CBD has potent anti-inflammatory qualities. THC is immunosuppressive at very high doses. At low doses, it can offer benefits as an analgesic and anti-inflammatory treatment.

Mindfulness Meditation Exercises

Before beginning any of the meditations, please bring kind awareness to:

- why you chose this topic
- how your belly, chest, and head each feel when you reflect on this topic
- the emotions that you can associate with these visceral feelings
- the positive or negative impact of any ideas you believe in regarding this topic
- when you can apply increased mindfulness to this topic in your day-to-day life

Access free audio version of these meditations at https://www.deirdramartinez.com/freemeditations

Sitting Meditation

Step 1: Arriving

Become still wherever you are—either lying, sitting, or standing, choose a posture to be as comfortable as possible, then lightly close your eyes.

Bring your awareness to whatever is going on for you right now.

Give the weight of your body up to gravity. Allow your weight to sink into the points of contact between your body and the floor, chair, or bed, whether that's your feet, your buttocks, or your back.

What sensations are there, right now? If you notice any tension or resistance to painful or unpleasant sensations, gently turn toward them. Accept them as best you can. If you begin to tense around the breath, then let go a little bit with each out-breath. Soften into gravity.

Notice any thoughts as they arise and pass away in the mind. See if you can let them come and go without becoming too identified with their content. Look at your thoughts, not from them. Observe them as if they were clouds in the sky. Relate to them as a flow of mental events. Remember, thoughts are not facts.

Notice any feelings and emotions as they arise. Can you let these come and go without pushing away those that you don't like, or jumping onto those that you do like? Include everything within your awareness with a kindly perspective.

Step 2: Gathering

Allow your awareness to gather around the experience of the breath in the body. Drop your awareness inside the breath and feel the different sensations in the front, back, and sides of the torso, inside the torso, and on the surface of the torso. Feel all of the different sensations of the breath as it flows into and out of the body.

Can you rest within the flow of the breath? Let everything change, moment by moment. Use the breath to anchor your awareness in the present moment and the body. Each time you notice your mind has wandered, remember that you are having a magic moment of awareness. You have woken up. Then gently bring the mind back to the breath deep in the body.

Step 3: Expanding

Gently broaden and expand your awareness to include the whole body. Feel the weight and shape of the body as it sits, stands, or lies. Feel the breath in the whole body. Imagine you are breathing in and out in all directions: 360-degree breathing.

If you have any pain or discomfort, make sure your awareness stays open to include this with a sense of compassion. Soften tension and resistance with each breath. Cultivate acceptance for all of your experience. Befriend it.

Now broaden your awareness even further to become aware of sounds both inside and outside the room. Be aware of other people around you.

Then imagine expanding all of your awareness outward to include all humanity. Imagine the whole world breathing.

Now gently open your eyes and move the body.

As you re-engage with the activities of your day, see if you can carry the awareness that you've cultivated with you.

Short Body Scan Exercise

Let's begin by taking a moment to allow your body to settle into a comfortable position. You may close your eyes or keep them slightly open, allowing the spine to lift, the shoulders to soften (5 seconds).

Today we will practice a short body scan, checking in with our bodies helps to settle the mind and to notice what physiological sensations and emotions might be present (2 seconds).

Begin by taking a full breath in and a long breath out (5 seconds).

Now bringing awareness to the top of your body, your head, face, neck, shoulders (3 seconds).

Noticing any sensations, movements, any places of holding (5 seconds).

Now moving down to the arms and the hands (5 seconds).

Sensing the back of the body, the front of the body (3 seconds).

Sensing yourself seated. Feeling the contact of your body with the chair or the cushion (10 seconds).

Now sensing your upper legs, your lower legs, and the feet (5 seconds).

Noticing if there are any particular places that call out for attention. Places where sensations feel most vibrant or dynamic (10 seconds).

Scanning to see if there places where there is a lack of sensations or only very faint sensations (5 seconds).

Now sensing the whole-body breathing (2 seconds). One complete organism (20 seconds).

Finishing with a full deep breath in and a long breath out (20 seconds).

Loving Kindness Meditation

Sit comfortably in a quiet place where you can be free from distractions.

Hold your spine neutral and tall.

Let your hands rest comfortably in your lap.

Close your eyes, or gaze softly at the earth ahead of you.

As you breathe slowly in and out through your nose.

Spend some time with attention on breath.

Without forcing, gently nudge your way into a longer inhale breath, and a much longer exhale breath.

Let the breath get quieter as your body softens a bit and your mind, too, gets quieter.

(pause for three to five breaths)

And now, at the center of your heart,

Imagine a source of radiant, soft, warm white light

The light is alive, vibrating, pulsing

Feel the light with your body

Its warmth, its movement, its energy

It's the limitless source of love, positivity, and wellbeing within you and because it is limitless, you can share.

Invite before you someone with whom you'd like to share this light

Someone you know. Someone you care for. Someone you love.

Sit them directly across from you.

They are sitting just as you are.

Their spine tall and neutral.

Their hands in their lap.

You can see them breathing, you can sense the rise and fall of their chest.

And now because you love this person so much,

You decide to send them four wishes,

As you send them your light.

You say silently to yourself:

May this person have happiness and all the causes of future happi-ness.

As you send them this wish, you also imagine light, traveling across all space and time from your body to theirs - filling them up with light.

(pause for three to five breaths)

And then you say to yourself:

May this person be free from their pain and suffering, and all the causes of their pain and suffering.

And as you send them this wish, you equally send them more light. The light now filling their entire torso with wellbeing.

(pause for three to five breaths)

And then you say to yourself:

May this person never be separated from joy. May they always be immersed in joy, never touched by pain.

Again, imagining more light sent over with this wish. The light has now filled up their arms and their legs.

(pause for three to five breaths)

And the you say to yourself:

May this person live always in a state of contentment, free from all of their grasping, and free from aversion.

And as you send over more light with this wish, it fills up their neck, it fills up their head.

Their entire body is now glowing with light.

(pause for three to five breaths)

Because of all the well wishes you sent, your loved one, your friend, is now glowing.

You see them, having received your wishes, and you understand that they are happy, free from pain, joyful and content.

Their light is so bright that it bounces back to you.

Your own light, now, even brighter.

Rest now, in the presence of this light.

And rest in the sensation in your body.

How does it feel, to see your friend, so happy and so free?

Recognize that it's by sharing with others, that we experience fullness.

Recognize that you are whole, you are perfect, and you have everything that you need.

Mindful Eating Exercise: Raisin Meditation

Place a few raisins in your hand. Imagine that you are a young child who is seeing this raisin for the very first time.

Now, with this food in hand, you can begin to explore it with all of your senses.

Scan it, exploring every part of it, as if you've never seen such a thing before. Turn it around with your fingers and notice what color it is.

Notice the folds and where the surface reflects light or becomes darker.

Next, explore the texture, feeling any softness, hardness, coarseness, or smoothness.

While you're doing this, if thoughts arise such as "Why am I doing this weird exercise?" "How will this ever help me?" or "I hate these raisins." Are you anticipating eating the raisin? Is it difficult not to just pop it in your mouth?

Then just see if you can acknowledge these thoughts, let them be, and then bring your awareness back to the raisin.

Take the object beneath your nose and carefully notice the smell of it.

Bring the object to one ear, squeeze it, roll it around, and hear if there is any sound coming from it.

Begin to slowly take the raisin to your mouth and let it touch your lips, noticing how the arm knows exactly where to go. Notice any sense of urgency and perhaps become aware of your mouth watering.

Place the raisin in your mouth and notice any sense of urgency. Breath and allow the raisin to move in your mouth before you start to chew. Become aware of what the tongue is doing. When you're ready, begin to chew the raisin slowly.

When you feel ready to swallow, consciously notice the intention to swallow, then see if you can notice the sensations of swallowing the raisin, sensing it moving down to your throat and into your esophagus on its way to your stomach.

CHAPTER 4 – SHINING THE SPOTLIGHT ON A BUDDING INDUSTRY

In the budding cannabis industry, every state that has legal access has their own challenges. In California, big business has big influence with big budgets for marketing. In addition, taxes are high (about 30 percent in California). Illegal black-market shops (that pay no taxes) are still operating, making it harder for legal dispensaries to profit. Dispensaries need extra cash flow and they turn to brands with big marketing budgets to buy shelf space to get products in front of the consumer. Unfortunately, it's becoming a pay-to-play game that isn't necessarily providing the best product for the client. The industry and market are constantly evolving, and consumers need to know how to rise above the chaos and make the best decisions for themselves.

Here is what you need to know to help you navigate the cannabis industry as a consumer.

1. Hemp vs. Marijuana CBD

Hemp CBD has less than .3 percent THC which is not enough to be psychoactive. For that reason, it is accessible nationwide. Marijuana CBD can have different ranges of THC from .4 percent - 30 percent, and psychoactivity will vary depending on the amount of THC, the individual's biochemistry, and tolerance. Marijuana CBD can only be purchased in a licensed dispensary (or illegal shops, but you don't want to buy from there -- more on that soon). There are therapeutic benefits to THC and opting for less than .4 percent may not be enough to provide that total wellness benefit.

The entourage effect is highly therapeutic and results from all the cannabinoids working together. Marijuana CBD provides the "full spectrum" of cannabinoids, whereas hemp CBD provides "broad spectrum," which has little to no THC. Lastly, cannabis is a phytoremediator which means that it absorbs toxins from the soil. Hemp CBD doesn't have the same regulation standards as the marijuana CBD that is sold in legal dispensaries. Hemp CBD companies are not required to test their products for contaminants, toxins, or ingredients. A study published by JAMA found that 26 percent of the products they tested contained less CBD than labeled, which could negate any potential clinical response.[53] Marijuana CBD is highly regulated and tested, in many cases making it cleaner than food!

2. The CBD industry's explosive growth is quickly outpacing science

Since the Farm Bill was passed in 2018, hemp became legal to grow throughout the United States. Hemp CBD is now found in a variety of products including body lotions, face creams, water, tinctures, and gummies. Prior to 2018, very little research was conducted on hemp because it was classified as a Schedule 1 Drug, which made it illegal. Now that hemp is legal, scientists are able to conduct the research needed to support the health claims many of these products promote. In the meantime, many of the claims being promoted by products are based on anecdotal accounts.

As of May 2020, the only confirmed medical condition that CBD treats effectively is epilepsy.[29] As cannabis becomes legalized throughout the country, there will be more research available and is currently underway for treating depression, anxiety, insomnia, and more.

3, Indica, sativa, hybrid, Oh My!

One of the first questions a budtender (a staff member who works at a dispensary) will ask is "Are you looking for an indica, sativa, or hybrid?"

They can usually see the confusion on the customer's face and then they'll realize they have a newbie in the shop, so the next question is usually, "How do you want to feel?"

That's easy! People turn to cannabis to spark their creativity, to calm their nerves, to help them sleep, to find pain relief, and more. Depending on how you want to feel, Budtenders will suggest different strains in either indica, sativa, or hybrid. Each strain has a different chemical profile of phytocannabinoids and terpenes (the chemical compounds in plants that provide smell, taste, and effect similar to essential oils). These profiles provide effects that in general are:

- Indica - Calming, Sleep inducing, and Relaxing
  - Popular Strains: Northern Lights, Skywalker
- Sativa - Stimulating, Creativity, and Energizing
  - Popular Strains: Jack Herrer, Blue Dream
- Hybrid - Mix of both Indica & Sativa
  - Popular Strains: Gelato, GG#4

There is so much cross breeding of plants now that most strains are hybrids. Also, these are generalizations, as each individual's body chemistry will have an impact on the effect. For example, indica doesn't always make me sleepy. Actually, I prefer to have an indica strain right before my yoga practice.

To lessen the confusion, many brands are starting to move away from strain names and opt for effects based labeling. For example, instead of looking for an Indica strain like Northern Lights, you can find a product labeled as "Calm." Currently, brands like Canndescent and Lola Lola provide this type of labeling, which make it much easier for new consumers.

4. Vapegate

In 2019, the Federal Drug Administration and Center for Disease Control made a statement warning consumers to not smoke THC vaping products amid an ongoing investigation into lung illnesses. Vapes are very popular because they are discrete, there is no odor and no butane lighting. They are also perceived as safer than smoking flower because the vapor doesn't have butane contaminants that could be found when smoking flower from a joint, pipe, or bong.

When this statement was released, vape sales plummeted. Consumers were afraid. What the media and FDA failed to reveal was that these products that were associated with the lung diseases were all purchased in the illegal market. After testing the products used by the patients who got sick, they discovered a common additive Vitamin E Acetate, which was used as a cutting agent, allowing illegal manufactures to alter the product to look like it had more cannabis oil but, in reality, it had less. No vape cartridges that were purchased in legal dispensaries had this additive and were not linked with any of the illnesses.

5. Be aware of the illegal market

Illegal marijuana dispensaries are very active in some states like California. In states where there is no legalization, the "black market" may be a friend you can call to get a new vape. In any case, buying from the illegal market is playing with fire. Products purchased in the illegal market are not tested for contaminants or toxins. As mentioned earlier with vaping, many products are manufactured with cutting agents or additives.

The problem is not only the risk to your health, but also that a lot of these illegal dispensaries do not look illegal at all. What is even more deceiving are illegal delivery services that are easily found online. Here are a few steps to take to ensure you're getting your cannabis from a legal trusted resource.

- Legal dispensaries have a Bureau of Cannabis Control license posted usually near the entrance. Don't be afraid to ask and see it. You can even look on their website beforehand and they'll have their license number posted online.
- If it looks shady, it probably is! Are Budtenders serving you cannabis from large jars instead of selling it prepackaged? Are they giving you free cannabis or letting you smoke in the shop? These are just a few clues that the shop is not legal.
- Use governmental agencies to verify licenses. In California, CApotcheck.com provides information about legal dispens-

aries near you.

6. Cannabis and The War on Drugs are social justice issues

The Great Depression of the 1920s left our country looking for a scapegoat. People of color were seen as a threat in the highly competitive job market. Cannabis was popular among minorities with roots in the Black jazz communities and Mexican farmers.

Harry Anslinger was the founding head of the Federal Bureau of Narcotics (FBN), a precursor to the Drug Enforcement Administration (DEA). He was known for producing racist and false propaganda. He attacked jazz musicians because this music scene created a first in American culture with white youth idolizing Black artists on a large scale. In a testimony to US Congress to support the Marihuana Tax Act of 1937 Anslinger states, "There are 100,000 total marijuana smokers in the US, and most are Negroes, Hispanics, Fillipinos, and entertainers. Their Satanic music, jazz and swing, result from the marijuana usage. This marijuana causes white women to seek sexual relations with Negroes, entertainers and any others." Louis Armstrong, the jazz musician who promoted cannabis use as a relaxant that "makes you forget all the bad things that happen to a Negro" was arrested for possession in 1930.

Hispanics were also a threat as immigration increased as a result of the Mexican Revolution (1910-1920). Mexicans used cannabis both medicinally and recreationally. Anslinger teamed up with William Randolph Hearst (newspaper tycoon) and pharmaceutical companies to launch an anti-marijuana campaign to profit off of manufactured medicine and deport thousands of Mexicans. It was during this time that anti-drug zealots swapped the term "cannabis" for "marihuana" or "marijuana," hoping that the Spanish word would conjure anti-Mexican sentiment. Newspapers ran headlines like "Mexican menace" or "marijuana menace."

The Controlled Substance Act of 1970 initiated the scheduling of drugs by how dangerous they were *perceived* to be. Marijuana was made a schedule 1 drug, which meant it had no accepted medical use and a high potential for abuse. In 1972, the DEA was founded with strict mandatory jail sentences for possession of drugs. Today, minority communities are still disproportionately affected by drug laws. Marijuana use is roughly equal among Blacks and Whites, yet Blacks are 3.73 times as likely to be arrested for marijuana possession.[54]

The government has a history of using scapegoats to deflect from bigger issues related to racism. With the recent development of cannabis as a pharmaceutical drug Epidiolex[29], there is no longer a debate on the medicinal properties. Cannabis must be reclassified and removed from Schedule 1 status. Non-profit organizations like The Last Prisoner Project, are dedicated to assisting those incarcerated from Marijuana related offenses. Check out the great work they're doing at www.lastprisonerproject.org.

Choosing cannabis exercises our freedom to self-medicate responsibly. I want to highlight responsibly. The opposition is still very strong and looking for any opportunity to take that freedom away. Responsible use is very similar to consuming alcohol and includes:

1. Not driving or operating heavy machinery while under the influence of cannabis
2. Being cautious of mixing cannabis with other intoxicating substances like alcohol
3. Purchasing legal cannabis
4. Not giving cannabis (THC) to minors
5. Starting with a low dose
6. Avoid consuming in public places. If you choose to, use something discreet like a vape or edible.

CHAPTER 5 - MYTHS & MISTAKES

Our perception is greatly influenced by our culture, social circles, family, and media. There are messages that circulate within our society about what is acceptable while rejecting anything that doesn't fit the norm or status quo. With internet especially, there is an overwhelming amount of information available that it is hard to decipher what is fact and what is fiction. It's easier to believe the myths rather than do the research. The common myths about cannabis are propaganda and hurtful. They create stigmas that shame people from exploring cannabis as complementary medicine.

Myth 1: Cannabis is a gateway drug

I remember when my mom found my first homemade pipe. It was a crushed Coca-Cola can that I carelessly tossed in the trash. It was the 1990s and there was a War on Drugs. She flipped because the propaganda was "cannabis is a gateway drug." Her fear was rooted in her experience with my father, who was a drug addict. She was obviously afraid I would turn out the same way. However, if anything was a gateway for me, it was McDonalds. By the time I was 8 years old, I was eating 20-piece chicken McNuggets super-sized meals and I was almost 200 pounds by the time I was 13. Food can be abused and be just as harmful as hard drugs on the street. People are dying from diet-related diseases every day. The problem is not the substance itself. If cannabis were really a gateway drug, then anyone who had ever tried it once would be a hardcore heroin addict. That's just not true. According to an article published by the National Institute of Health, "The majority of people who use marijuana do not go on to use 'harder' substances."[55]

The real problem is the pain that the person is numbing with the drug. As addiction expert Dr. Gabor says, "We need to stop asking 'why the addiction?' and start asking 'why the pain?'" Using cannabis as a scapegoat distracts us from the real issue which is that people are in pain. They use substances to numb the pain and it works, even if it's only temporary relief. What we really need to do as a society is help heal the trauma and pain that is causing one to escape with substances.

Myth 2: Cannabis causes weight gain

This is only half true. Cannabis can cause the munchies if not used appropriately. THC can stimulate hunger. However, a study published in the Journal of Epidemiology found that long term use of THC may actually have the opposite effect.[56] How? Let's take a closer look at the endocannabinoid system, composed of ECBs like Anandamide and 2 AG plus Cannabinoid receptors (CB1 and CB2) located throughout the body. CB1 receptors are found in the brain and nervous system, as well as in the peripheral organs and tissues, and are the main target of THC.

In this study, researchers hypothesized that repeated CB1 receptor stimulation from THC use can lead to desensitization of its effects. Similar to caffeine, we can build a tolerance to THC. When the eCBs our body makes like 2-AG bind to CB1 receptors, it releases appetite stimulating hormones… hello, munchies! However, continued cannabis use leads to an oversaturation of THC preventing 2-AG from binding to CB1 receptors eventually suppressing appetite.

Munchies are more likely to happen with recreational users as they only occasionally consume THC and haven't developed enough THC in their system to block 2-AG from binding to CB1 receptors.

A few ways to prevent the munchies include microdosing (taking small amounts of about 2mg of THC throughout the day). A side effect of THC use is dry mouth. Thirst can often be mistaken for hunger. Try drinking water before reaching for the bag of chips.

Myth 3: The Higher the THC, The Higher the Experience

Back in the 70s, Cannabis was Sungrown. It was cultivated out-doors, in the natural elements, organically, and the THC content was no more than 5%. As cultivation methods improved, THC content increased. Whereas today with indoor cultivation, the environment can be manipulated to help produce THC content as high as 40%.

To the average consumer, the perception that a higher THC per-centage will get you higher is a myth that is driving prices in the marketplace. Due to consumer demand, flower that is 25.5% THC or more can sell for $60-$80 for an 1/8th of an ounce! That's like $20 a joint! There is also speculation and investigation, in some cases, on the legitimacy of these potency claims. Some companies have been fined for misrepresenting THC content in order to boost sales.

What actually does effect the level of "high" one experiences comes from "the entourage effect." The combination of all the different cannabinoids and terpenes. Each strain has it's own unique profile. Because cannabis is a crop, each batch will also have a range in cannabinoid makeup. For example, you may buy Alpine Blue Dream indoor flower testing at 25% and then buy it again at the same store a few weeks later but now it's testing at 22% THC (because it's from a new different batch). When you smoke it, the difference may be subtle. You may even find that the lower THC gets you higher!

I remember experiencing this firsthand at a smoke lounge in Palm Springs, The 420 Lounge. The dispensary was a client and they offered me a joint by Henry's Original. I asked for something with low THC because I still had a 2 hour drive home. The joint was only 11% THC but I was floored! I ended up staying at the lounge a few hours until I sobered up. Luckily, it was drag queen bingo night so I was highly entertained.

Myth 4: Cannabis is a cure-all

I love cannabis for its therapeutic benefits, but therapeutic doesn't mean cure. We have to remember that healing is a mental, emotional, physical, and spiritual process. There are amazing drugs that do help people overcome diseases. However, we cannot depend on substances to heal us. Real healing is a journey that is complex and critical to the evolution of consciousness. Dependency on outside substances shadows the spiritual gifts that lie inside. Illness sparks a wakeup call that there is a disconnection from wholeness and balance. Cannabis is a plant medicine that is an ally, not a savior. Only you can save yourself.

In many native cultures, spiritual practitioners such as shamans, curanderos, and medicine men use plant medicine in their healings. Plants, specifically any psychedelic, are very powerful substances. Guides offer support in plant medicine journeys thereby lessening the likelihood of having a negative experience or developing a substance dependency. It is best practice to work with a holistic practitioner trained in plant medicine to support you in your journey. Their guidance will help you get to the root of what is causing your health problem rather than just putting another Band-Aid on.

Cannabis is complex and it's easy to make mistakes. Don't let that deter you from exploring it's therapeutic potential. Here are some of the most common mistakes and how you can prevent a negative experience.

Mistake 1: Dosing

All too often, I hear horror stories about edibles making it difficult for consumers to trust cannabis again. The challenge is that everyone's biochemistry is different, and some individuals are more sensitive to THC. Five milligrams of THC may feel like nothing to one individual, while it may make another individual high for the next 24 hours.

The best way to navigate dosing is to start low and go slow. Look for products with 2mg or lower and also include CBD since CBD has a balancing effect with THC. When CBD is added to a product containing THC, it can minimize any paranoia or anxiety which can be a side effect from THC sensitivity. When ingesting cannabis, wait 45 minutes to an hour in order to feel the effect and before taking more. The effects from ingestibles also tend to last longer, so be prepared for an experience to last 2-4 hours. Sublingual strips may have a faster reaction time. Smoking cannabis by vape or flower provides the fastest effects, usually within a few minutes.

When in doubt, keep a journal to track your dosing, product, and effect. If you prefer digital, I recommend the app Releaf that you can download from the Apple store for free.

Mistake 2: Stigma

Stigma is defined as a set of negative beliefs that a group or society holds about a group of people or topic. Stigma is a shaming or mark of disgrace. It is rarely based on facts, but rather on preconceptions and generalizations.

Culturally, there is a huge stigma around mental health and drug users. You may hear cannabis users referred to as "stoners" or "pot heads' ' which are negative stereotypes. Stigma results in prejudice, rejection, and discrimination. People that hold these stereotypes believe that shame can force people to conform with their beliefs, but that is simply not the case. It has the opposite effect, perpetuating more discrimination, and preventing people from utilizing alternative medicine like cannabis.

Recovery is not linear and there are different paths. For some, cannabis is actually part of their recovery from addiction to more harmful drugs like opioids. A method called harm reduction re-places a lethal addictive substance with a less harmful substance. Abstinence may be too extreme for some and harm reduction pro-vides another way to ease into recovery.

Lastly, the stigma of cannabis users being unproductive, low-life "stoners" is just not true. Here is a list of successful celebrities who openly consume cannabis:

- Lady Gaga (musician)
- Wille Nelson (musician)
- Snoop Dog (musician)
- Sarah Silverman (comedian)
- Seth Rogan (actor/producer/comedian)
- Melissa Ethridge (musician/breast cancer survivor)
- Woody Harrelson (actor/comedian)

Mistake 3: CBD can still show up on a drug test

There's just enough THC in cannabis CBD (not Hemp derived) that if you're using it on a regular basis, like taking capsules every day, the THC can build up in the liver and thus eventually into your bloodstream and can skew a drug test. This is a big reason why we need the laws changed. People who want to use CBD for strictly therapeutic purposes (no psychoactivity) are limited if their employer does drug testing. Cannabis needs reclassification and removal as a Schedule 1 drug.

There are drug test kits that people swear help you remove any trace of cannabis use. I've never used them and therefore can't recommend any. Do your research and if you do decide to use one, then do a test run before your actual drug test.

Mistake 4: Buyer conformity

Although cannabis has been used as medicine for thousands of years, it is only recently being sold as a commodity. It is a new industry with a lot of big business trying to dominate the market.

There is also white-labeling happening all the time, meaning the same product will be in different brands, with different labels, and different prices, but it really is the same product inside. The price may be higher in one brand because it has a more popular name. You're basically paying extra to support their marketing budget rather than for a better quality product.

Consider what you value as a customer rather than going for a popular brand. Questions to ask yourself are:

- Does the brand support small farmers?

- Does the product use organic ingredients?

- Is the product's lab results third party tested? Is it lab tested at all?

- Is the product made in small batches for optimum freshness?

- Does the brand support the community?

- Does the brand provide consumer education and resources?

- Does the brand provide consistent quality?

- Is the brand minority owned?

- Does the brand have healthy options like Vegan? Sugar Free?

Mistake 5: Lack of support

When someone is new to using cannabis therapeutically, they can make the mistake of using the wrong products for their desired effect, getting too "high," not consuming enough Cannabinoids to get the desired effect, not being consistent with dosing, and not making the lifestyle adjustments to complement their treatment. This can all be prevented with the help of a trusted guide or expert.

Even if you're someone who consumed cannabis recreationally for years, using it therapeutically to treat health conditions is a completely different ballgame. The reason is because the real therapy is coming from a holistic model. Consuming cannabis by itself will only address the symptoms. In cannabis therapeutics, we're getting to the root of what is causing physical, emotional, and mental pain. There are deeper core issues like trauma or habitual self-sabotaging behavior that need to be elevated and healed. It also takes time to find your therapeutic threshold which often requires tracking your experience for several weeks.

Lastly, nutrition, exercise, and stress management will have a great impact on the long-term benefits of cannabis therapeutics. Without addressing those lifestyle changes, consumers could develop a cannabis dependency.

CHAPTER 6:
CASE STUDY

Laurey was a student of my Zumba class for years. When she mentioned to me, she had been having problems with anxiety and depression, I offered to work with her in cannabis therapeutics.

Laurey is a professional businesswoman who works in accounting and is married with two adult children. In her late 50s, she is experiencing early stages of menopause and has a very healthy lifestyle that helps manage the symptoms. However, she started experiencing anxiety and depression that left her feeling fatigued for days. She hated how it interfered with her quality of life and relationships. In the middle of the day at work, she would have a panic or depressive episode that made it impossible to be productive at work.

She went to see her doctor, who placed her on antidepressants and she also started working with a therapist. Although she started to feel better for a short time, about six months later, she started having suicidal thoughts and digestive upset. When she went back to her doctor to explain what was happening, the doctor wanted to prescribe even more medication. That's when she knew she needed an alternative.

Another doctor she had seen had told her that CBD might be helpful. She started using a CBD vape pen and noticed some relief. She was having a positive experience with the vape pen, but still had bouts of depression and suicidal thoughts. When she found out that I had a cannabis therapeutics program, she was very interested and signed up, hoping I could introduce her to other products and guide her through the healing process using cannabis as an alternative treatment to her prescription pills.

She saw her enrollment in my program as an investment and committed fully. She showed up to all the coaching sessions, she did all her growth work, and even did yoga which she'd previously resisted. She'd always been put off by yoga because she said, "I'm too tight and can't sit still." However, because of her commitment, she decided to ignore her inner critic and did the yoga anyway. Eventually, she fell in love with yoga.

She explains:

"The program changed the way I see yoga. Before, I did not like it at all. Deirdra taught me how to take deep breaths that helped me relax throughout the day. She sent several videos teaching me how to use

yoga to work through depression. I learned how to slow down and take breaks. Now I like yoga and practice at least three times a week. After practicing I feel very calm."

Laurey learned how to use yoga and mindfulness meditation to help manage her episodes of depression. When she noticed herself feeling a episode coming on, she used the tools she learned in our program to overcome them quickly. Eventually, she stopped having panic attacks and suicidal thoughts. She also found new cannabis products that worked even better for her than the vape she initially used. Cannabis became a supplement to the deeper work she did in healing the disconnection she had between her mind, body, and breath.

"Now I feel much better, with a lot less stress. I used to take pills for depression, which of course had side effects. Now I am not taking them anymore. Yes, my life has been improved, I used to have panic episodes quite often. These episodes used to take me hours to recover, but now I have them very sporadically and I recover very fast from them," Laurey adds.

CHAPTER 7: TAKE YOUR RESULTS TO A HIGHER LEVEL

Over 10 years of fitness training and helping women transform their bodies, I learned that the best results came from those that made a commitment to a program or working with a coach. I've had many consultations with women who expressed years of trying every diet, or reading every weight loss book, or attending various workshops. They had some success, but never achieved the long-term transformation they hoped for.

This is not different when you look at any sort of transformation program. There were a few common excuses and concerns they all shared that prevented them from achieving their optimum health. These may be similar blocks preventing you from living your best life!

1. I don't have enough money
2. I don't have enough time

3. What if I don't succeed?

Health as wealth

Cheap does not equate to transformative results. Watching free talks and doing free workouts on YouTube is a great resource. However, there is no accountability, no customization, and no support. I could learn a lot by reading a book from Tony Robbins, but I'd get a completely different experience and impact from going to one of his live events or even working with him directly. Most of us probably can't afford to hire Tony Robbins directly, but there are qualified coaches at a more affordable price that can walk you through your journey. Cannabis therapeutics is highly specialized because we're looking for someone who has experience in nutrition, fitness, stress management, and cannabis. It will save you time and energy in the long term if you work with an experienced practitioner.

Health restoration is priceless. Feeling energized, uplifted, and centered can bring out the best in productivity, relationships, and creativity. With optimal health, how much more money could you make? How much more present could you be with your loved ones? If you're single, how much more confident would you feel to date? What ends up costing more is workout equipment or gym memberships that never get used, health foods and dietary supplements that never get eaten because they taste like cardboard.

When taking care of your health is fun, effective, and customized, you're not only going to enjoy the experience, but the results will also last long term.

Time is valuable

How do you really spend your time? How much do you watch TV? How much time do you spend on your laptops or mobile devices mindlessly searching the web or social media? How much time is spent unproductively? Think about the amount of distractions you're bombarded with every second. Are you able to stay focused?

I once heard this quote in a personal development course, that we all have the same amount of time. It's not like some people are blessed with more time than others. We all have the same amount of hours in the day. It depends on how we choose to spend those hours. The way we prioritize our time is different.

Time is valuable because we don't get it back. Once it's spent, it's gone. If we lose money, we can always make it back. With time, we don't have that opportunity.

Therefore, it's important to be efficient with our time. We can't expect our health and happiness to improve if we're not putting time into it. Taking time to prepare healthy meals, meditate, exercise, stretch, walk outside, and self-care is vital to our livelihood. If it feels like there is no time in the day, then we need to do some purging and restructuring.

Take an honest look at the way you spend your time. If you've developed habits of mindless searching through TV, social media, or the internet, then stop! You don't have to stop completely, just designate a specific amount of time to engage in that activity. For example, if you use social media for business purposes, you may need to schedule one or two hours a day versus someone who uses it to stay connected to friends and may only really need 15 minutes a day.

It doesn't have to stop there. Think about other habits that take up a ton of your time. At one point, my eating disorder took up a ton of my time. I was constantly looking for a perfect diet, shopping and preparing meals for those diets. Then I spent an inordinate amount of time thinking about food or my body. I realized that my obsession over food and body was just another distraction. If I didn't have a food and body "problem" I needed to fix, then what else could I be doing? When I decided to drop the diet drama, I made more time in my life for the projects that I really wanted to work on.

Spiritual teacher Marianne Williamson said, "Our deepest fear is not that we are inadequate. Our deepest fear is that we are powerful beyond measure. It is our light not our darkness that most frightens us." Use time wisely, as an instrument of our own power. You get to decide how to use your time, so make it count. Prioritize what you value most.

Conviction wins

Believing in yourself and your body's innate ability to heal itself is incredibly therapeutic. In the study of epigenetics, we learn that science is proving that our bodies ability to heal and repair itself is greatly affected by our beliefs, thoughts, emotions, and intentions. Everything is energy. When we don't have faith in our own ability, then the body shuts down. We create our own reality through the mind, body, and spirit connection. If we want a better life, we need to think more highly of ourselves, our circumstances, and others. As epigenetics expert Dr. Bruce Lipton says, "Your perception of any given thing, at any given moment, can influence the brain chemistry, which, in turn, affects the environment where your cells reside and controls their fate."

Pay attention to the language you use to talk about yourself. Do you use self-deprecating language like, "I shouldn't have done that," "What's wrong with me?" "Why can't I get this right?" Whether these words are said out loud or stay in your head, they have a physiological impact. These messages put the body into a stress response mode causing the "fight, flight, or freeze" activation of our nervous system. The body's reaction is protection from a perceived threat.

To quote *Dr. Lipton again,* "Our beliefs control our bodies, our minds, and thus our lives…"

CHAPTER 8 - A HIGHER STATE OF HEALTH

The main point to bring home here is that a higher state of health is holistic and evolutionary. To achieve wellbeing, there is no magic pill or plant that can independently heal you. Health and wellness result from bringing balance to our physical, mental, emotional, and spiritual bodies. Naturally, they work interdependently and synergistically. It's when one of these bodies is impaired that illness or health issues become problematic.

When any cannabis product promises to "cure" a particular health issue, take it with a grain of salt. Keep in mind that there is something very powerful—the mind—that can trigger the placebo effect. This means that if you believe something works, it will. The product itself may not have enough cannabis to truly have an impact, but the belief that it will work may actually promote positive effects.

The mind is that powerful in healing and with that takes great responsibility. Stress starts in the mind and can wreak havoc on the body. Develop a practice of stress management through yoga and meditation to learn how to calm the mind and release tension from the body. Work with a therapist or personal development coach to help break free from limiting beliefs.

Learn how to process emotions in a constructive way rather than distracting or suppressing them. Emotions can trigger chemicals in the body that can either promote or reduce stress. It's important to work with our emotions in a way that we can harness their energy. Become aware of your emotional states and how they are in constant flux throughout the day. Use breathing exercises and meditations to help with managing them. Have a support circle of friends you can trust as well as an outlet like a journal to express yourself freely. Movement is also a great outlet for emotional release or stimulation.

Healing is a spiritual evolutionary process. Disease, illness, and health challenges are all symptoms of spiritual disconnection. We've lost ourselves and forgotten who we really are. The journey of health and healing is a spiritual homecoming. A remembering of the wholeness and love that is always within.

As hippie dippie as that all sounds, it works. It's time to get out of our heads and into our hearts. Worry, shame, guilt, resentment, and anger are all thought-based energies that can create chronic stress in the body. Love, compassion, empathy, and understanding are all heart felt energies that promote healing and restoration.

Cannabis is a tool to help us restore homeostasis in the body while we work on the deeper issues of what is causing the imbalance. Are there lifestyle habits to change? A healthier mindset to adopt? Emotions to be processed? Do we need to love ourselves? Love our bodies?

Not addressing the root of what is causing the imbalance can lead to cannabis dependency or the complete opposite where cannabis has no therapeutic effect at all. The root of our pain can either be a source of self-imprisonment or a seed of transformation. It takes a conscious choice to work with our pain instead of avoiding it.

Root down to rise up and take your health to a higher level with cannabis therapeutics. Enjoy the journey!

REFERENCES

1 McFarlane, A. The long-term costs of traumatic stress: intertwined physical and psychological consequences. *World Psychiatry.* 2010; Feb; 9(1): 3–10.

2 Substance Abuse and Mental Health Services Administration (SAMHSA, 2018) *Key Substance Use Indicators in the United States: Results from the National Survey on Drug Use and Health*

3 Brand, J and Zhongzhen, Z. Cannabis in Chinese Medicine: Are Some of the Traditional Indications Referenced in Ancient Literature Related to Cannabinoids? *Frontiers in Pharmacology.* 2017; 8: 108.

4 American Psychological Association. (2007, October 24). *Stress a Major Health Problem in The U.S., Warns APA.* Retrieved from: https://www.apa.org/news/press/releases/2007/10/stress

5 American Psychological Association. (2017, November 1). *Stress in America, The State of our Nation.* Retrieved from: https://www.apa.org/news/press/releases/stress/2017/state-nation.pdf

6 US Department of Health & Human Services (2019, March 14). *Office of Women's Health. Stress and Your Health.* Retrieved from https://www.womenshealth.gov/mental-health/good-mental-health/stress-and-your-health#2

7 Farooq, K., Williams, P. Headache and chronic facial pain. *Continuing Education in Anaesthesia, Critical Care & Pain.* 2008; 8(4): 138–142.

8 Substance Abuse and Mental Health Services Administration (SAMHSA) Center for Behavioral Health Statistics and Quality. (2018). 2017 National Survey on Drug Use and Health: Detailed Tables. Table 8.56A (PDF, 36.1 MB).

9 SAMHSA. (2013). Table 4: *Specific mental illness and substance use disorders among adults, by sex: percentage*, United States, 2001/2002. Behavioral Health, United States, 2012. HHS Publication No. (SMA) 13-4797. Rockville, MD: Substance Abuse and Mental Health Services Administration.

10 Vaccarino, V., Shah, A.J., Rooks, C., Ibeanu, I., Nye, J.A., Pimple, P., et al. Sex differences in mental stress-induced myocardial ischemia in young survivors of an acute myocardial infarction. *Psychosomatic Medicine*. 2014; 76(3): 171–180.

11 Grundmann, O., Yoon, S.L. Irritable bowel syndrome: epidemiology, diagnosis and treatment: an update for health-care practitioners. *Journal of Gastroenterology and Hepatology*. 2010; 25(4): 691–699.

12 Michopoulos, V. Stress-induced alterations in estradiol sensitivity increase risk for obesity in women. *Physiology & Behavior*. 2016; 166: 56–64.

13 Louis, G.M., Lum, K.J., Sundaram, R., Chen, Z., Kim, S., Lynch, C.D., et al. Stress reduces conception probabilities across the fertile window: evidence in support of relaxation. *Fertility and Sterility*. 2011; 95(7): 2184–2189.

14 Hamilton, L.D, Meston, C.M. (2013). Chronic Stress and Sexual Function in Women. *Journal of Sexual Medicine*. 2013;10(10): 2443–2454.

15 Dennerstein L, Dudley EC, Hopper JL, Guthrie JR, Burger HG. A prospective population-based study of menopausal symptoms. *Obstet Gynecol*. 2000; Sep; 96(3):351-8.

16 Nosek M, Kennedy H, Beyene Y, Taylor D, Gilliss C, Lee K. The

Effects of Perceived Stress and Attitudes Toward Menopause and Aging on Symptoms of Menopause. *Journal of Midwifery Women's Health.* 2010; Jul-Aug; 55(4): 328–334.

17 Shahbadeh, M (2019). *US Diets and Weight Loss - Statistics and Facts.* Retrieved from: https://www.statista.com/topics/4392/diets-and-weight-loss-in-the-us/

18 Garner, D.W., Wooley, S.C. Confronting the failure of behavioral and dietary treatments for obesity. *Clinical Psychology Review.* 1991;11, pp. 727-780.

19 Harrop, E. N., & Marlatt, G. A. The comorbidity of substance use disorders and eating disorders in women: prevalence, etiology, and treatment. *Addictive Behaviors.* 2010; 35, 392-398.

20 Mangweth, B., Hudson, J. I., Pope, H. G. Jr., Hausmann, A., DeCol, C., Laird, N. M., ... Tsuang, M.T. Family study of the aggregation of eating disorders and mood disorders. *Psychological Medicine.* 2003; 33, 1319-1323

21 Altman, S. E., & Shankman, S. A. What is the association between obsessive-compulsive disorder and eating disorders? *Clinical Psychology Review.* 2009; 29, 638-646.

22 American Psychological Association (2012). *Inappropriate Prescribing.* Retrieved from: https://www.apa.org/monitor/2012/06/prescribing

23 Howie LD, Pastor PN, Lukacs SL. Use of medication prescribed for emotional or behavioral difficulties among children aged 6-17 years in the United States, 2011-2012. *NCHS Data Brief.* 2014 Apr; (148):1-8.

24 Vowles KE, McEntee ML, Julnes PS, Frohe T, Ney JP, van der Goes DN. Rates of opioid misuse, abuse, and addiction in chronic pain: a systematic review and data synthesis. *Pain.* 2015;156(4):569-576.

25 National Institute of Health (NIH) (2020). Opioid Overdose Crisis. Retrieved from: https://www.drugabuse.gov/drugs-abuse/

opioids/opioid-overdose-crisis#six

26 Hill A.J., Williams C.M., Whalley B.J., Stephens G.J. Phytocannabinoids as novel therapeutic agents in cns disorders. *Pharmacology & Therapeutics.* 2012; 133:79–97.

27 Alger, Bradley. Getting High on the Endocannabinoid System. *Cerebrum,* 2013;14.

28 Mechoulam R., Sumariwalla P.F., Feldmann M., Gallily R. Cannabinoids in models of chronic inflammatory conditions. *Phytochemistry Reviews.* 2005; 4:11–18.

29 United States Food & Drug Administration. (2018, June 25). *FDA approves the first drug comprised of an active ingredient derived from Marijuana to treat rare, severe forms of epilepsy.* Retrieved from: https://www.fda.gov/news-events/press-announcements/fda-approves-first-drug-comprised-active-ingredient-derived-marijuana-treat-rare-severe-forms

30 Carrie Cuttler, Alexander Spradlin, Ryan J. McLaughlin. A Naturalistic Examination of the Perceived Effects of Cannabis on Negative Affect. *Journal of Affective Disorders,* 2018; Aug 1; 235: 198-205

31 Izzo A.A., Borrelli F., Capasso R., di Marzo V., Mechoulam R. Non-psychotropic plant cannabinoids: New therapeutic opportunities from an ancient herb. *Trends Pharmacology Science* 2009; 30:515–527.

32 Carlson L. E. (2012). Mindfulness-based interventions for physical conditions: a narrative review evaluating levels of evidence. *ISRN psychiatry, 2012,* 651583. https://doi.org/10.5402/2012/651583

33 McPartland JM, Guy GW, Di Marzo V. Care and Feeding of the Endocannabinoid System: A Systematic Review of Potential Clinical Interventions that Upregulate the Endocannabinoid System. Romanovsky AA, ed. *PLoS ONE.* 2014;9(3):e89566.

34 Dietrich A, McDaniel WF Endocannabinoids and exercise. *British Journal of Sports Medicine* 2004 Vol 38 (5)

35 Sparling PB, Giuffrida A, Piomelli D, et al. Exercise activates the endocannabinoid system. *NeuroReport*. 2003;14 :2209–11.

36 Smolen J.S., Burmester G.R., Combeet B. NCD Risk Factor Collaboration (NCD-RisC) Worldwide trends in body-mass index, underweight, overweight, and obesity from 1975 to 2016: A pooled analysis of 2416 population-based measurement studies in 128.9 million children, adolescents, and adults. *Lancet*. 2017; 390:2627–2642.

37 Donovan A. Argueta, Nicholas V. DiPatrizio. Peripheral endocannabinoid signaling controls hyperphagia in western diet-induced obesity. *Physiology & Behavior*. 2017; 171: 32

38 Pagano C1, Rossato M, Vettor R. Endocannabinoids, adipose tissue and lipid metabolism. *Journal of Neuroendocrinology*. 2008 May;20 Suppl 1:124-9.

39 Bosch-Bouju, Clémentine, and Sophie Layé. "Dietary Omega-6/Omega-3 and Endocannabinoids: Implications for Brain Health and Diseases." Cannabinoids in Health and Disease. *InTech*, 2016.

40 di Tomaso, Emmanuelle. "Brain cannabinoids in chocolate." *Nature* 382 (1996): 677-678.

41 Hassanzadeh P, Hassanzadeh A. The CB1 receptor-mediated endocannabinoid signaling and NGF: the novel targets of curcumin. *Neurochemical Research*. 2012; 37: 1112–1120.

42 Stith, S.S., Vigil, J.M., Brockelman, F. *et al.* The Association between Cannabis Product Characteristics and Symptom Relief. *Sci Rep* **9**, 2712 (2019)

43 Yann Le Strat, Bernard Le Foll. Obesity and Cannabis Use: results from 2 representative national surveys. *Journal of Epidemiology*. 2011; Oct 15; 174(8):929-33

44 Melissa Prud'homme, Romulus Cata, Didier Jutras-Aswad. Cannabidiol as an Intervention for Addictive Behaviors: A Systematic Review of the Evidence. *Substance Abuse.* 2015; 9: 33–38.

45 Li X, Vigil JM, Stith SS, Brockelman F, Keeling K, Hall B. The effectiveness of self-directed medical cannabis treatment for pain. *Complementary Therapies Med.* 2019;46:123-130.

46 Institute of Medicine (US) Committee on Advancing Pain Research, Care, and Education. *Relieving Pain in America: A Blueprint for Transforming Prevention, Care, Education, and Research.* Washington (DC): National Academies Press (US); 2011.

47 Bohnert AS, Ilgen MA, Galea S, McCarthy JF, Blow FC. Accidental poisoning mortality among patients in the Department of Veterans Affairs Health System. *Med Care.* 2011;49(4):393-396.

48 Centers for Disease Control and Prevention. *2018 Annual Surveillance Report of Drug-Related Risks and Outcomes — United States. Surveillance Special Report 2.* Centers for Disease Control and Prevention, U.S. Department of Health and Human Services. Published August 31, 2018. Retrieved from: https://www.cdc.gov/drugoverdose/pdf/pubs/2018-cdc-drug-surveillance-report.pdf?s_cid=cs_828

49 Bachhuber MA, Saloner B, Cunningham CO, Barry CL. Medical Cannabis Laws and Opioid Analgesic Overdose Mortality in the United States, 1999-2010. *JAMA Intern Med.* 2014;174(10):1668–1673.

50 Elikkottil, J., Gupta, P., & Gupta, K. (2009). The analgesic potential of cannabinoids. *Journal of opioid management, 5*(6), 341–357.

51 Black, D. S., & Slavich, G. M. (2016). Mindfulness meditation and the immune system: a systematic review of randomized controlled trials. *Annals of the New York Academy of Sciences, 1373*(1), 13–24.

52 Nagarkatti, Prakes, et all. Cannabinoids as novel anti-inflam-

matory drugs. *Future Medicine Chemistry*. 2009 Oct; 1(7): 1333–1349.

53 Marcel O. Bonn-Miller, PhD, Mallory J. E. Loflin, PhD, Brian F. Thomas, PhD, Jahan P. Marcu, PhD, Travis Hyke, MS, and Ryan Vandrey, PhD Labeling Accuracy of Cannabidiol Extracts Sold Online. *Journal of the American Medical Association*. 2017 Nov 7; 318(17): 1708–1709.

54 American Civil Liberties Union (ACLU) Report: *The War on Marijuana in Black and White: Millions of Dollars Wasted on Racially Biased Arrests*. 2013. Retrieved from: https://www.aclu.org/report/report-war-marijuana-black-and-white?redirect=criminal-law-reform/war-marijuana-black-and-white

55 National Institute of Health in Drug Abuse (2017) *Letter from the Director on Marijuana* Retrieved from: https://www.drugabuse.gov/publications/research-reports/marijuana/letter-director

56 Le Foll, Trigo JM, Sharkey KA, Le Strat Y. Cannabis and Δ9-tetrahydrocannabinol (THC) for weight loss? Medical Hypotheses. 2013 May;80(5):564-7

If you enjoyed this book, please take a moment
to leave a positive review.

Thank you!

www.ingramcontent.com/pod-product-compliance
Lightning Source LLC
Chambersburg PA
CBHW070812240726